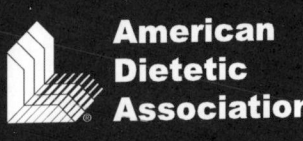

American
Dietetic
Association

D1793430

Spanish

for the

Nutrition
Professional

Peggy A. Batty

Contributing Editor: Mary Jo Kurko, MPH, RD

Diana Faulhaber, Publisher

Jason M. Muzinic, Acquisitions Editor

Elizabeth Nishiura, Production Editor

10 9 8 7 6 5 4 3 2 1

Library of Congress Cataloging-in-Publication Data

Batty, Peggy A.
  Spanish for the nutrition professional / Peggy A. Batty; contributing editor, Mary Jo Kurko.
    p. ; cm.
  Includes bibliographical references.
  ISBN 0-88091-406-8
    1. Spanish language—Conversation and phrase books (for nutritionists)

[DNLM: 1. Nutrition—Phrases—English. 2. Nutrition—Phrases—Spanish. 3. Diet—Phrases—English. 4. Diet—Phrases—Spanish. 5. Health Education—methods. 6. Hispanic Americans—ethnology.] I. Kurko, Mary Jo. II. American Dietetic Association. III. Title.

PC4120.N87B38 2005
468.3'421'0246132—dc22

                                        2004026338

Table of Contents

Acknowledgments

I would like to thank Beth Vinkler, Julie Moreschi, Julie Davis, Catherine Arnold, and Becky Baumann of Benedictine University for their help and encouragement with this project; all the students who have taken the Spanish for Nutrition Professionals course and contributed their ideas; and my daughters, Tara and Robin, for helping me put my original book together.

I also thank Jason Muzinic for his interest in this project and his persistence in seeing it through, and Mary Jo Kurko for all her help and her sparkling enthusiasm.

—*Peggy A. Batty*

I would like to thank Frances Rich and Leslee Ala for encouraging me with this and many other projects and Jason Muzinic of the American Dietetic Association for sharing his knowledge and expertise and for his infinite patience. I am grateful for the unwavering support of my daughters, Maggie and Annie. They have not only read hundreds of nutrition materials for me but also eaten experimental recipes, carried bag lunches that were portioned into "proper servings," and used sanitizing solution without complaint!

I would also like to thank Aldo Arellano and Jose Luis Tapia Guzman for answering my questions and correcting my accent and Kathi Goehring for trusting my professional judgment.

—*Mary Jo Kurko, MPH, RD*

Reviewers

Ana Eugenia Blanco
Sodexho Mid-Atlantic Dietetic Internship, Rockville, MD

Digna Cassens, MHA, RD
Country Villa Health Services, Marina Del Rey, CA

Jennifer Christensen, RD
Utah Valley Regional Medical Center, Provo, UT

Luis A. Corado, RD
Harbor-UCLA Medical Center, Torrance, CA

Jean Tiffany Cox, MS, RD
University of New Mexico School of Medicine, Albuquerque, NM

Maria Figueroa, RD
Davita Decatur Dialysis, Emory-Adventist Hospital, Decatur, GA

Marilyn Figueroa, EdD
Nutrition Consultant, Teaneck, NJ

Illia Fontanez-Cowles, RD, MS
North Florida Regional Medical Center, Gainesville, FL

Melissa Franz, MPH, RD
Hidalgo County WIC Program, Edinburg, TX

Jacqueline Gomes, RD
Union Hospital, Union, NJ

Cynthia M. Goody, PhD, RD
University of Cincinnati Medical Center, Cincinnati, OH

Myriam Grajales-Hall
University of California, Agriculture and Natural Resources, Riverside, CA

Catherine Held, RD
St. Margaret Mercy—ARAMARK, Hammond, IN

Sylvia E. Melendez-Klinger, MS, RD
Hispanic Food Communications, Hinsdale, IL

Debbie Polisky, MS, CLE
Clinica Adelante, Surprise, AZ

Cynthia Seline Sanchez, RD
Hidalgo County WIC Program, Edinburg, TX

Kelli L. Schenk, RD
Brummit and Associates, Hennessey, OK

Martha A. Schofield, RD
South Carolina Department of Health and Environmental Control, Pee Dee Public Health District, SC

Michele Silano, MA, MS, RD
Diet Experts, LLC, Bergenfield, NJ

Milton Stokes, RD
Sodexho—North General Hospital, New York, NY

Poppy Strode, MS, MPH, RD
California Department of Health Services, WIC Branch, Sacramento, CA

Samantha Wiggins, RD
St. Margaret Mercy—ARAMARK, Hammond, IN

Foreword

A fellow Spanish-speaking dietitian practicing in Texas shared a humorous counseling experience. She was reviewing a list of fish products high in n-3 fatty acids with a Spanish-speaking patient from Colombia and noticed that the patient giggled when they discussed sardines (*sardinas*). When asked why she was giggling, the patient explained that in Colombia teenage girls are often referred to as *sardinas*. The obvious message is that Latinos may speak Spanish but not all words mean the same thing in different cultural subgroups.

Now more than ever, Spanish-language nutrition education materials are necessary to better serve the rapidly growing Spanish-speaking population in the United States. Nutrition professionals must recognize this rapid change and prepare themselves to meet the challenge of successfully communicating nutrition education messages to this population.

Spanish-language nutrition education materials must be culturally appropriate and reflect the diversity of Latino culture. To avoid embarrassing situations, such as the one described at the opening of this Foreword, it is important to ask publishers and authors whether their materials are intended for specific cultural subgroups. Another important task is to inquire about the reading level of Spanish-language materials. Translated materials (from English to Spanish) must be assessed for reading literacy in Spanish to ensure that they are appropriate for a specific population.

As nutrition professionals try to decide whether specific materials are appropriate for the cultural groups they serve, it helps if they have some knowledge of the Spanish language. *Spanish for the Nutrition Professional* is a great first step for anyone wanting to take on the challenge of studying the Spanish language to improve communication with Spanish-speaking clients. Spanish-language skills will help keep the lines of communication open between the nutrition practitioner and the client and their family.

Of course, effective communication involves more than just speaking a common language. One must also consider the cultural factors of the population being served. The first section of this book provides an excellent overview of Latino culture. This section and the "cultural tidbits" interspersed in other sections of the book keep the nutrition professional connected with important information about Latino culture.

The American Dietetic Association is commended for publishing this valuable resource. Nutrition professionals who use *Spanish for the Nutrition Professional* to improve their communication skills in Spanish and to learn more about Latino culture will find it to be a worthwhile pocket guide.

Delia Solis, MS, RD

Chair, Hispanics in Dietetics and Nutrition (HIDAN)
A Networking Group of the American Dietetic Association

"HIDAN functions as a resource for health professionals who provide Hispanic communities with food and nutrition services and/or education."

2003–2004 Board

Chair: Delia Solis, MS, RD

Co-chair: Carmen Roman-Shriver, PhD, RD

Secretary: Cecilia P. Fileti, MS, RD, FADA

Treasurer: Carina Roe-Saez, RD, CDE

Newsletter: Judith C. Rodriguez, PhD, RD, FADA

ADA Liaison: Claudia M. Gonzalez, MS, RD

Section I

Culturally Sensitive Nutrition Care of the Spanish-Speaking Client

Chapter 1

Latino Culture

Hispanic/Latino Diversity

The term "Hispanic" is an ethnic category that denotes neither race nor color, and a Hispanic may be white, black, or American Indian. Although the term is widely used, many members of the Hispanic population prefer the term "Latino." The U.S. Census Bureau considers the terms interchangeable as of January 1, 2003 (1).

Despite the unifying Spanish language and cultural similarities, there is tremendous variety within the Latino community. Latinos are stereotypically thought of as Mexicans (in California, Texas, Illinois, and Arizona), as Puerto Ricans (in New York, New Jersey, and Pennsylvania), or as Cubans (in Florida). However, the group "Latinos" also includes persons from Central and South America, as well as individuals in the Southwest who were born in the United States but whose ancestors are Spanish (1).

According to the 2000 Census, Hispanics/Latinos comprise about 12.5% (35.3 million individuals) of the US population. (This number excludes 3.8 million residing in the Commonwealth of Puerto Rico.) Latinos are the largest minority group in the United States. Only 3% of the dietetics profession is Hispanic/Latino, and counseling Latino clients can be a challenge for nutrition professionals (2). Most dietitians will be counseling members of a cultural group that differs from their own (3).

Basic Cultural Issues

To provide appropriate care to Latino clients, nutrition professionals must understand Latino culture. Although there are differences among Spanish-speaking cultures, similarities include the Spanish language, importance of family, and religious faith (4).

The Latino family may include parents and children, as well as grandparents, cousins, aunts and uncles, godparents, and close family friends. The father is often the "head of the family," and the mother is usually responsible for the home. Family members feel responsibility for other family, especially for those with health problems. Therefore, it is not unusual for family members to accompany the client to nutrition counseling. If this is the case, keep in mind that it is not unusual for the father to make health decisions for other family members (5).

Religion may be another factor for the nutrition professional to consider in the decision-making process. The church (more than 90 percent of all Latinos are Catholic) is often part of daily family and community life and plays an even greater role in times of illness (5).

Although most Latinos speak Spanish, there are numerous dialects. Individuals from different countries (or areas of the same country) may not give the same meaning to a particular word. Despite the differences in vocabulary, most Spanish-speaking Latinos have no difficulty conversing with each other. Young people who have been raised in the United States commonly use a mix of Spanish and English.

Difficulty in accessing and using the health care system in the United States (especially for Latinos of lower socioeconomic status) is a significant health problem. Language barriers, a low rate of medical insurance coverage, the lack of transportation to and from clinics and hospitals, and low incomes are just a few factors that contribute to difficulty accessing services (4).

Potential Differences among Cultural Groups

In her publication *Community Nutrition in Action*, Marie Boyle (6) lists areas of potential differences among cultural groups that nutrition professionals should consider in a cross-cultural nutrition counseling session. Some of these differences are as follows:

- *Socioeconomic and environmental factors.* Socioeconomic issues (including legal status) and environmental risks can affect health and treatment and can influence a client's attitudes, beliefs, and values.

- *Language.* New immigrants are likely to speak Spanish only. Furthermore, many Latinos who speak and understand English cannot read or write English.
- *Family structure and social values.* Western medicine makes a person responsible for his or her health care. The Latino culture of extended family invites (especially the head of the household) collective decision making. Strong traditional gender roles (for example, the mother being responsible for cooking and feeding the family) may cause women to perceive the changes suggested in nutrition counseling more negatively (7).
- *Cultural food practices.* Food behaviors (such as food preferences, preparation, eating patterns, and foods used for medicine or to promote health) that are reflective of the Latino culture are most evident in recent immigrants, but some cultural behaviors persist for generations.
- *Health care values, beliefs, and practices.* Although Western cultures rely on science to explain illness and treat disease, some Latino cultures focus more on the spiritual causes of illness.
- *Attitudes toward health care providers.* Some Latino groups (especially men) may feel that seeking medical attention is a sign of weakness. Latinos may seek a health care provider's assistance only after a disease has progressed—not for preventive care or for natural processes like pregnancy. Also, some Latinos may use home remedies for an illness before visiting a doctor (6).

References

1. US Department of Commerce. The Hispanic population: Census 2001 brief. Issued May 2001. Available at: http://www.census.gov/prod/2001pubs/c2kbr01-3.pdf. Accessed March 6, 2004.

2. Rogers D. Report on the ADA 2002 dietetics compensation and benefits survey. *J Am Diet Assoc.* 2003;103:243–255.

3. Curry K, Jaffe A. *Nutrition Counseling and Communication Skills.* Philadelphia, Pa: WB Saunders; 1998.

4. Kemp C. Mexican and Mexican-Americans: health beliefs and practices. Available at: http://www3.baylor.edu/~Charles_Kemp/ hispanic_health.htm. Accessed January 26, 2004.

5. Clutter A. Understanding the Hispanic culture. Ohio State University fact sheet. HYG-5237-00. Available at: http://ohioline.osu.edu/hyg-fact/5000/5237.html. Accessed February 17, 2004.

6. Boyle M. *Community Nutrition in Action*. 3rd ed. Belmont, Calif: Wadsworth Publishing; 2003.

7. Kittler P, Sucher K. *Food and Culture in America*. 2nd ed. New York, NY: Van Nostrand Reinhold; 1997.

Chapter 2

Folk Beliefs, Lay Healers, and Other Treatments in the Latino Culture

Although Latinos may use folk or home remedies to treat illness, they likely also use (sometimes simultaneously) antibiotics and other medications. Furthermore, Latinos may believe that health, in general, is a matter of fate, and therefore may feel little responsibility for seeking treatment. They may give almost equal weight to physical and psychosomatic illness (1).

Understanding cultural beliefs is essential to provide appropriate nutrition counseling. In fact, what may be most important to your Latino clients is not your education and training, but the manner in which you provide your nutrition counseling (1).

Hot/Cold Theory

Latinos of Mexican and Puerto Rican descent may subscribe to two folk illnesses that could have nutritional implications: the hot/cold theory and *susto* (soul loss). In the hot/cold theory, balancing hot and cold foods and conditions is a part of maintaining good health (1,2).

"Hot" and "cold" properties are assigned to foods and conditions, but not everyone classifies specific foods and conditions the same way. Generally, "hot" conditions are related to vasodilation and high metabolic rate. For example, pregnancy, hypertension, diabetes, and acid indigestion are usually considered "hot" conditions (3,4). On the other hand, "cold" conditions involve vasoconstriction and low metabolic rate. Examples of a "cold" condition might be headache, earache, or stomach cramps (4).

Based on the hot/cold theory, a "hot" condition would require a "cold" treatment to restore balance, whereas a "cold" condition calls for "hot" herbs and foods. Chili peppers, garlic, onion, most grains, and tuna fish are examples of "hot" foods, whereas "cold" foods usually include vegetables, tropical fruits, dairy products, and white fish. Beans and food made of corn, rice, or wheat, as well as foods high in sugar, are deemed hot or cold depending on how they are prepared (4).

Keep in mind that Latinos who follow folk beliefs, such as the hot/cold theory, may avoid sharing their beliefs with health care providers (3). Use careful, indirect questions to find out if your client believes in such theories. Working with your client's individual hot/cold food beliefs will increase satisfaction and compliance with the nutrition care plan (5,6).

Soul Loss

Susto (soul loss) is a condition believed to be the result of the soul escaping from an individual's body. Some Latinos believe that a number of diseases (including cancer, kidney failure, diabetes, and high blood pressure) are a result of *susto*. This belief can be part of a Latino client's reluctance to consult health care providers for treatment (1). As with the hot/cold theory previously discussed, knowing that your client subscribes to *susto* can help you develop a culturally appropriate nutrition care plan.

Lay Healers

The first treatment step for some Latino clients might be a home remedy, such as a tea made from various herbs or spices. If such treatments are ineffective, advice from an herbalist or a massage therapist could be sought (1).

After the home remedy or herbalist, the next step could be to consult a *curandero* (lay healer). The *curandero*, through a combination of spiritualistic and Western medicine, seeks to treat the physical and psychological aspects of illness. *Curanderos* are not used (or are not reported as used) as often in the United States. This may be due to increased use of Western care with acculturation, or use may simply be underreported (1).

Far more Latinos use physicians as primary sources of health care than lay healers. Be aware, however, that a client may simultaneously use prayer, folk and/or herbal remedies, and prescription medications (1).

Herbal Remedies and Other Treatments

Herbs are often used for disease treatment in many cultures. Many herbal remedies are harmless, and there is evidence of efficacy for some herbal treatments. However, ingredients in herbal preparations may interact with medications, and some herbal remedies are dangerous (3). As with all clients, the nutrition professional should probe for specifics if herbal remedies are being used.

Commonly used herbs that are safe for most clients include garlic (for yeast infections in the mouth, toothache pain, and stomach disorders); oregano (for fever and dry cough); chamomile (for colic, menstrual cramps, and insomnia); boiled peanut broth (for diarrhea); eucalyptus (for bronchitis); peppermint (for dyspepsia); and aloe vera (for burns) (3,4).

Unsafe treatments include *azarcón* and *greta*, which are lead-based and mercury-based products. (These treatments may be used for gastrointestinal conditions.) The traditional honey-and-water cure for infant colic should be avoided because of the risk of infant botulism (4). Unsafe herbs include aconite, belladonna, borage, chaparral, comfrey, ephedra, germander, kava, kombucha, lobelia, pokeroot, sassafras, skull cap, and wormwood (3,7). Be sure to consult a pharmacist or a reputable herbal text for guidance if you are unsure about a specific herb your client is taking.

References

1. Culture-sensitive health care: Hispanic. In: *From What Language Does Your Patient Hurt In? A Practical Guide to Culturally Competent Care*. Amherst, Mass: Diversity Resources; 2000. Available at: http://www. diversityresources.com/rc04_sample/hispanic.html. Accessed January 27, 2004.

2. Martinez RA. *Hispanic Culture and Health Care: Fact, Fiction, and Folklore*. St. Louis, Mo: Mosby; 1978.

3. Kemp C. Mexican and Mexican-Americans: Health beliefs and practices. Available at: http://www3.baylor.edu/~Charles_Kemp/ hispanic_health.htm. Accessed January 26, 2004.

4. Kittler P, Sucher K. *Food and Culture in America*. 2nd ed. New York, NY: Van Nostrand Reinhold; 1997.

5. Boyle M. *Community Nutrition in Action*. 3rd ed. Belmont, Calif: Wadsworth Publishing; 2003.

6. National Alliance for Hispanic Health. A primer for cultural proficiency: Towards quality health services for Hispanics. Washington, DC: Estrella Press; 2001. Available at: http://www.hispanichealth.org/pdf/primer.pdf. Accessed March 6, 2004.

7. Boyle MA, Anderson SL. *Personal Nutrition*. 5th ed. Belmont, Calif: Wadsworth Publishing; 2003.

Chapter 3

Differences in Dietary Habits Within the Latino Community

Latino Dietary Habits and Staple Foods

A knowledge and understanding of cultures and ethnic food practices is essential in providing appropriate nutrition counseling. Understanding the factors that impact a client's decision-making process allows the nutrition professional the opportunity to implement permanent behavior change rather than simply "prescribing a diet" (1).

General nutritional concerns for Latino clients include the following:

- High fat intake (sometimes in the form of lard), which may offset the benefits of a diet high in vegetable protein and carbohydrates from beans and rice or beans and corn tortillas
- Few servings of green or leafy vegetables and milk
- A diet high in sugar, including sweetened beverages
- Increased incorporation of fast food as acculturation occurs (2)

In many Spanish-speaking countries, a light meal is served for breakfast (*desayuno*). The main meal of the day is lunch (*almuerzo, comida,* or *lonche*). *La merienda* or *entrecomidas* is a light snack (mostly for children), which may be served in the early evening. In the late evening, a small supper (*cena*) is served (3). As acculturation occurs, most Latinos adopt the three-meals-a-day (with the heavier meal in the evening) pattern of the United States.

Although food preparation and practices can change slowly for Latinos once they arrive in the United States, some practices (such as fast food), may be adopted quickly. Change depends on the community, availability of native foods, family income, and the length of time the family has lived in the United States. It is very individual (4).

Mexican Foods

Staple foods of Mexican-American families (especially those with limited incomes) include beans, rice, and tortillas. Corn or flour tortillas, if homemade, are small, and five to ten may be eaten at a meal. Tortillas are eaten in the home; bread is usually eaten away from home. Pinto beans, black beans, garbanzo beans, and kidney beans are very popular and may be served several times every day. Beans may be boiled for breakfast, fried for lunch, and refried for the evening meal. Rice may be prepared in soup with vegetables and/or meat, or served with vegetables in which all the water has been steamed out (the rice may be fried in oil before the water is added) (5).

Protein foods include eggs, cheese, beef, pork, chicken, turkey, shrimp, red snapper, and other firm-fleshed fish. Many Mexican foods that are stuffed (for example, tacos, enchiladas, tamales, quesadillas, and burritos) have become staples in the United States as well.

Vegetables are usually part of a dish, not served separately. Some common choices include cactus, carrots, chilis, corn, cucumber, jicama, onions, peas, potatoes, radishes, squash (chayote, pumpkin, summer), squash blossoms, tomatillos, tomatoes, and yucca. Hearty soups or stews are popular choices for dinner.

Common semitropical and tropical fruits include avocados, bananas, cherimoya, coconut, granadilla, guava, lemons, limes, mangos, melon, cactus fruit, oranges, papaya, passion fruit, pineapple, plantains, strawberries, and *zapote* (fruit of the sapodilla tree). Many fruits are eaten in the form of *aguas*, pureed fruits with sugar added.

The most common traditional desserts are *arroz con leche* (rice pudding), *capirotada* (bread pudding), *buñuelos* or *sopaipillas* (fritters), flan, and *pan dulce* (similar to a large cookie).

Coffee with large amounts of sugar and milk is often preferred. *Atole* is a warm, milk-based beverage, flavored with chocolate, fruit, or nuts, and thickened with very finely ground *masa* (corn flour). Although natural fruit drinks are popular in Mexico, carbonated beverages are quickly incorporated into the diet once individuals are in the United States (5). Few dairy products are used—a segment of the population is lactose intolerant. Also, because tap water is unsafe in much of Mexico and Central America, new immigrants may need to be reassured that tap water is safe in the United States.

Food is often spicy (there are more than ninety varieties of chiles), but spicy sauces vary with the region of Mexico. In addition, seasonings such as anise, cilantro, cinnamon, cumin, cocoa, epazote (a pungent herb that is also called Mexican tea), garlic, mace, and vanilla are commonly used (5,6).

Puerto Rican Foods

Staple foods of Puerto Rican-Americans include rice, beans (often fried first, sometimes with oil added to the top at the end), especially kidney beans and *gandules* (pigeon peas). Garbanzos (chickpeas), navy beans, and black-eyed peas are also common. *Viandas*, a group of starchy tubers, which are frequently used before they ripen, are also staple foods (6). Common *viandas* include the following:

- *Arracachá*
- Breadfruit
- Cassava (manioc, yucca)
- *Tanier* (white, yellow)
- Taro (dasheen, malanga)
- Unripe banana
- Potato
- Yam (orange, white)
- Ripe plantain
- Sweet potato (yellow, white)

An *arracacha* looks something like a white carrot and tastes like carrot, celery, and cabbage mixed; a ripened banana is a fruit, not a *vianda*. For more information about these vegetables and other traditional Latino cuisine, see Raichlen's *Healthy Latin Cooking* (7) or consult one of the many helpful online resources available.

Popular fruits and vegetables include avocados, bananas, beans, cashew apples (the fruit surrounding the cashew nut), coconuts, guavas, mangos, papayas, passion fruit, pineapple, soursop (*guanábanana*), several types of squash (including chayote), and tomatoes.

Fish is more plentiful than meat. One of the most popular kinds of fish is *bacalao* (codfish). *Bacalao* can be eaten fresh or dry and cured with salt. Note that a client who is following a sodium-controlled diet should not regularly eat *bacalao* that is cured in salt. Other common fish include bonito, grouper, mackerel, salmon, red snapper, and tuna (5).

Sofrito is a seasoning sauce made by sautéing diced peppers, onions, garlic, cilantro, annatto seeds, and spices with pieces of fried pork or pork sausage. It may contain tomatoes (especially in Cuban cuisine) and can be purchased already prepared.

Café con leche, strong coffee with hot milk and sugar, is a popular beverage and may also be served to children. It is not a foamy drink and is usually three-quarters coffee. However, when prepared for children, more milk is usually added. Clients from the Dominican Republic may drink coffee made with sweetened condensed milk added.

Cuban Foods

Cuban food preparation and practices are similar to Puerto Rican. Staple foods of Cuban-American families include rice, beans (especially black beans), and *viandas*. Black beans that are cooked with rice are called *congri* (6). In El Salvador, it is called *casamiento* (which means "marriage").

Cubans eat many sweets made from fruits and *viandas*. A very popular and well-liked candy made from coconut is called *paneletas*.

References

1. Curry K, Jaffe A. *Nutrition Counseling and Communication Skills.* Philadelphia, Pa: WB Saunders; 1998.

2. National Alliance for Hispanic Health. *A Primer for Cultural Proficiency: Towards Quality Health Services for Hispanics.* Washington, DC: Estrella Press; 2001. Available at: http://www.hispanichealth.org/pdf/ primer.pdf. Accessed March 6, 2004.

3. Clutter A. Understanding the Hispanic culture. Ohio State University fact sheet. HYG-5237-00. Available at: http://ohioline.osu.edu/hyg-fact/5000/5237.html. Accessed February 17, 2004.

4. Warrix M. Cultural diversity: eating in America: Mexican-American. Ohio State University extension fact sheet. HYG-5255-95. Available at: http://ohioline.osu.edu/hyg-fact/5000/5255.html. Accessed February 14, 2004.

5. Kittler P, Sucher K. *Food and Culture in America.* 2nd ed. New York, NY: Van Nostrand Reinhold; 1997.

6. Syracuse CJ. Cultural diversity: eating in America: Puerto Rican. Ohio State University extension fact sheet. HYG=5257-95. Available at: http://ohioline.osu.edu/hyg-fact/5000/5257.html. Accessed March 19, 2004.

7. Raichlen S. *Healthy Latin Cooking.* New York, NY: Rodale Press; 1998.

Chapter 4

Establishing a Counseling Relationship

Creating a Positive Nutrition Counseling Relationship

Internationally known speaker and cross-cultural expert, Suzanne Salimbene, PhD, lists six keys for building a good professional relationship with Latino patients or clients (1). These are (*a*) show respect; (*b*) establish trust; (*c*) involve the family in decision making and care; (*d*) accept a different sense of time; (*e*) take pains to establish understanding and agreement; and (*f*) respect the spiritual side of physical complaints. Nutrition professionals can achieve these goals by using the following guidelines.

Respect

Show proper respect to your clients by greeting them (older adults first) formally, by title and family name. If you are uncertain about how to pronounce a name, be sure to ask. You should also refrain from using a client's first name at the beginning of a relationship (unless your client is a child). If you are speaking Spanish, use the formal *usted* rather than the informal *tú* for "you" (1).

Shake hands at the beginning of each meeting. A firm and slightly longer handshake is appropriate. Note that Latinos may show respect by avoiding eye contact with you; however, they will expect you to look directly at them. This remains true even if you are working through an interpreter (2).

Latino clients respect health care providers because of their healing abilities, education, and training. However, they will also expect to receive respect from you (1,2). In fact, being shown respect is so important to Latinos that your client may terminate the counseling relationship if he or she does not feel respected. For many Latinos, showing respect means not asking uncomfortable questions or expressing negative feelings, so you must gently encourage questions (2).

Trust

Take the time that your Latino client needs to establish trust. Oftentimes, Latino clients want a personal but not informal relationship with their health care providers. Although this may seem time-consuming, if trust is not established, a client may avoid conflict or confrontation with you by saying that he or she understands or by quickly agreeing to a treatment plan (2). On the other hand, if you have established a trusting relationship, your client may follow a treatment plan as a personal favor to you (1,3,4). Two techniques to personalize your approach and begin to establish trust with your client are (*a*) inquiring about the client and his or her family before asking more formal questions; and (*b*) letting clients know that they should tell you if they prefer not to answer any of your questions (5).

Family Involvement

Involve the family (especially those involved with food preparation) in the nutrition counseling session (1,2). (Because of regulatory issues and privacy concerns, you may want to respectfully obtain the client's written consent for the family members to accompany him or her and be possibly privy to confidential issues.)

Working with Interpreters

Interpreters and translators can help you provide effective nutrition counseling. Note that there is a difference between interpreters (who convert verbal languages) and translators (who work with written language).

If you do not speak Spanish or if your client has no English-language ability, using a trained interpreter who has expertise in the language and the culture of the client is best for both you and your client. Considering the Latino culture, an ideal interpreter would be older than your client and of the same gender (5).

Realize that if family members or friends are used as interpreters, your client may be reluctant to share certain concerns and it may be more difficult for you to assess your client's understanding. Although it is common to use children to interpret for parents, this practice should be a last resort because it places the parent and the child in a position of reversed power and authority. In general, it is best to have Spanish-speaking staff or volunteers interpret if a professional interpreter is not available (4). However, if staff are not familiar with medical terminology, they may unknowingly make mistakes.

The following are basic guidelines for the nutrition professional working with interpreters. Most of these guidelines are also appropriate for working with clients with limited literacy skills (1,2,5).

- Determine what questions you will ask before the counseling session begins.
- Be open to questions your client asks.
- Use open-ended questions, such as "Tell me how you . . . " rather than questions that can be answered with "yes" or "no."
- Learn a few words in your client's language (at least introductory greetings and good-byes.)
- Speak in short sentences and ask one question at a time. Interpreters may have difficulty converting long statements without forgetting something important. (Your client may also have difficulty following long sentences.)
- Avoid technical terminology, professional jargon, abstractions, and idioms and other expressions that would not be familiar to a nonnative English speaker.
- Make sure conversations are two-way (3), and look at and speak directly to your client, not the interpreter (5,6).
- Even though you do not understand the language, listen when your client speaks to the interpreter and look for nonverbal cues from your client.
- Schedule enough time. A session with an interpreter will take at least twice as long as usual.

- Have the interpreter ask the client to repeat the information that you have communicated to see whether your client understands. (This also allows the client to ask questions.) When doing this, it is important to request that the interpreter use your client's exact words, so that you can assess understanding more accurately (5).

Cross-cultural Communication

Communication and the relationship between you and your client are key to successful nutrition counseling. Successful counseling to the Latino client (and to most others, too) is not just technically accurate information, but also the way in which the counseling is provided (4).

Client-centered counseling emphasizes self-responsibility and the active participation of the client in designing a personal nutrition program. Some Latino clients may not respond well to this approach (3). Because the Latino culture often places the family's needs before the individual's, independence may not be valued. In addition, if clients feel powerless, they are less likely to believe that they can assume direct responsibility for their health (5).

It is essential to listen to your client's personal cultural beliefs rather than to assume that he or she reflects the stereotypical Latino culture. It is equally important to understand that your client's values and motivation are not necessarily the same as yours (3). For example, because of cultural values, Latino mothers may be pleased when their infants or children are overweight. Thus, they do not react as expected when the nutrition professional offers calorie-lowering suggestions.

To help your client feel more comfortable sharing his or her feelings, try to convey acceptance by using phrases like "I feel that . . . ." Speak slowly and clearly and in a conversational tone. Realize that raising the volume of your voice will not help your client understand—in fact, it is likely to be offensive (3).

Nonverbal Communication

Nonverbal communication is important in counseling all clients. As previously stated, some Latino clients may be reluctant to make their real attitudes known directly, and in such cases, nonverbal communication is even more important for counseling success.

Physical touch is the most personal form of nonverbal communication and thus, highly variable. Generally, a touch on the arm or brief pat on the shoulder is acceptable to clients whom you know (1,5).

Individuals tend to believe more of what they see than of what they hear, so body language is important with any client with whom you do not share a language. Try to convey warmth and acceptance with your body language (7).

Closed Gestures

If you hold your arms or books in front of your torso or your hand in front of your face, you are displaying a "closed gesture," hiding yourself from those facing you (7). This is considered negative.

Pointing

Pointing is acceptable if you need to point to a diagram or words on a paper. However, when you gesture toward your client, use your whole hand, not a pointing finger (7).

Seating

Because your shoulders signal where your interest is, lean slightly forward with your upper body facing toward your client when you are seating. When your client is speaking, move closer and listen carefully. The physical space between Latinos when holding a conversation may be closer than what you are accustomed to. If possible, have more than one chair, and let your client choose a seat (5,7). Some counselors and clients feel more comfortable angled toward each other instead of facing each other (7).

Facial Expressions

Avoid frowning because it may make your client feel that you are skeptical about what he or she is saying. This seems obvious, but many people frown while thinking about how to answer questions. Do not look over the rims or through the bottoms of your bifocals if you wear glasses. Although a few nods are affirming, excessive nodding can be perceived negatively (7).

Assessment of Health Beliefs and Practices

Medical anthropologist and noted cross-cultural expert Dr. Arthur Kleinman developed an interview tool that assists health care professionals to obtain information in a culturally unbiased manner (5). The questions are open-ended and will increase your clients' comfort level and help them to be more open to your counseling suggestions (5).

Following are a few of Dr. Kleinman's questions. Use your professional judgment to decide which of the questions to ask (5).

- What do you call this problem you are having? (Use the word[s] the client uses in place of the words "problem" and "it" in the next questions you ask.)
- What do you think caused this problem?
- Why do you think it started?
- What kind of treatment do you think you should receive?
- What are the most important results you hope to receive from treatment?
- How can I help you today?
- Is there anyone else in your family you'd like me to talk to?
- Have you seen a healer for this problem? Are you using the suggested treatment?

Culturally Sensitive Interviewing

Once you have gained some understanding of your client's beliefs, continue with the interview. Berlin and Fowkes developed a patient-centered approach (the LEARN tool) for culturally sensitive interviewing in 1983. Others have modified and added to the basic tool (5). The LEARN guidelines can help you negotiate a culturally sensitive nutrition treatment plan.

1. *Listen.* Use active listening to demonstrate that what your client has to say is very important to you and to help build your relationship.
2. *Explain.* To make sure you understand accurately, restate (explain) what you think your client said. Restating lets your client correct misunderstandings or explain further.
3. *Acknowledge.* First point out the similarities in what your client believes and what you feel is appropriate in the

cause and/or treatment of the problem. Then talk about the differences.

4. *Recommend.* Give your client options that are culturally appropriate and practical. Give the fewest options that still constitute proper nutrition care.

5. *Negotiate.* As with any client, after discussing the options, ask where the client would like to begin.

References

1. Culture-sensitive health care: Hispanic. In: *From What Language Does Your Patient Hurt In? A Practical Guide to Culturally Competent Care.* Amherst, Mass: Diversity Resources; 2000. Available at: http://www.diversityresources.com/rc04_sample/hispanic.html. Accessed January 27, 2004.

2. National Alliance for Hispanic Health. *A Primer for Cultural Proficiency: Towards Quality Health Services for Hispanics.* Washington, DC: Estrella Press; 2001. Available at: http://www.hispanichealth.org/pdf/primer.pdf. Accessed March 6, 2004.

3. Curry K, Jaffe A. *Nutrition Counseling and Communication Skills.* Philadelphia, Pa: WB Saunders; 1998.

4. Clutter A. Understanding the Hispanic culture. Ohio State University fact sheet. HYG-5237-00. Available at: http://ohioline.osu.edu/hyg-fact/5000/5237.html. Accessed February 17, 2004.

5. Boyle M. *Community Nutrition in Action.* 3rd ed. Belmont, Calif: Wadsworth Publishing; 2003.

6. Kemp C. Mexican and Mexican-Americans: health beliefs and practices. Available at: http://www3.baylor.edu/~Charles_Kemp/hispanic_health.htm. Accessed January 26, 2004.

7. Desmond P, Copeland L. *Communicating with Today's Patient.* San Francisco, Calif: Josey-Bass; 2000.

Chapter 5

Latino Health Profile

Notable Nutrition-Related Diseases in Latinos

The leading cause of death in Latinos is heart disease. Although cholesterol levels are similar to those in the non-Latino population, Latinos are less likely to know if they have high cholesterol levels. Furthermore, Latino men are more likely to have undiagnosed, untreated, or uncontrolled hypertension than non-Latino men (1).

Latinos (especially Mexicans and Puerto Ricans) are twice as likely as non-Latino whites to develop diabetes, and almost twice as likely to die from it (1). There is also a high prevalence of undetected diabetes in the Latino population.

Obesity is more common in Latinos (especially Mexican-American women) than in the general population. Thirty percent of Mexican-Americans are at a healthy weight, compared with 43 percent of non-Hispanic whites and 34 percent of non-Hispanic blacks (1).

Nutrition Concerns in Latino Children

Bottle-feeding is common among Puerto Ricans and some other Latino groups, partially because of bottle-feeding campaigns conducted in Latin America by corporations that market baby formula (1). Furthermore, where breastfeeding is practiced, there is a tendency to stop earlier and to introduce solid food earlier than current pediatric guidelines recommend (2).

Latino children eat less than the recommended servings of fruits and vegetables. After the age of 5 years, most Latino children do not get the recommended servings of milk each day (1), and as toddlers they tend to stay on bottles (containing milk and sweetened drinks) longer than is recommended.

Disease Prevention

Because disease prevention is not highly valued in some Latino cultures, Latinos have a higher prevalence of chronic illnesses. Lack of health insurance (more than one-third of the Latino population in the United States are uninsured) is another barrier to disease prevention. However, acceptance of health promotion and disease prevention concepts seems to be increasing, although interest in physical activity outside the context of manual labor remains low (1-3).

References

1. National Alliance for Hispanic Health. *A Primer for Cultural Proficiency: Towards Quality Health Services for Hispanics.* Washington, DC: Estrella Press; 2001. Available at: http://www.hispanichealth.org/pdf/ primer.pdf. Accessed March 6, 2004.

2. Culture-sensitive health care: Hispanic. In: *From What Language Does Your Patient Hurt In? A Practical Guide to Culturally Competent Care.* Amherst, Mass: Diversity Resources; 2000. Available at: http://www. diversityresources.com/rc04_sample/hispanic.html. Accessed January 27, 2004.

3. Kemp C. Mexican and Mexican-Americans: health beliefs and practices. Available at: http://www3.baylor.edu/ ~Charles_Kemp/hispanic_health.htm. Accessed January 26, 2004.

Chapter 6

Effective Communication

Communicating Nutrition Information to Latino Clients

The following specific guidelines will help you to communicate nutrition information to your Latino clients.

Language Skills

Some clients may not read or write Spanish or English and may need to bring a family member (who may or may not read Spanish or English) to the counseling session if a trained interpreter is not available. (Reminder: Because of regulatory issues and privacy concerns, obtain the client's written consent allowing family members to be present and to be privy to possibly confidential issues.) You should also have nutrition education materials (written in Spanish) that you feel comfortable using (1). Consider using actual food packages, food models, and measuring cups and spoons, because these tools may help clients with limited English-language skills (1,2).

Indirect Approach

A less direct approach may lower the risk of misunderstanding and hurt feelings. Make observations rather than judgments about behaviors. For example, try to say "people" rather than "you" when making comments (1). Use open-ended questions, such as "How do you cook your vegetables?" rather than a yes-or-no question such as "Do you cook your vegetables without salt?" (1,3).

Key Messages

Most people, including clients, do not speak the standard language of nutrition professionals. Therefore, focus on key messages (and essential skills and behaviors) rather than on information that may simply be nice to have (4).

Positive Food Practices

Although some clients may simply need guidance in selecting healthier foods, less acculturated clients may need help in modifying traditional foods or in learning to use available foods. In the *Journal of the American Dietetic Association*, Marian L. Neuhouser (5) recommends that nutrition professionals provide fat reduction information, especially to recent immigrants, and encourage Latino clients to *(a)* maintain high intake of fruits and vegetables, *(b)* maintain eating bread and potatoes without added fat, and *(c)* make modifications to traditional foods. For example, vegetables can be added to soups or stews; brown rice can be used instead of white rice; and green leafy vegetables can be added to salads (6).

Folk Beliefs

If a belief causes no harm, such as placing a safety pin over the abdomen of a pregnant woman to protect against the "evil eye," do not offer opinions of the practice. (See Chapter 2.)

Teaching and Learning Implications

As stated above, nutrition terminology is unfamiliar to the general public (4,7). Therefore, nutrition professionals need techniques to increase levels of understanding. Differences in educational levels and language skills directly affect understanding and comprehension (8,9). Although limited literacy does not mean limited intelligence or motivation, many clients who are ill, afraid, or under stress often have a lessened ability to understand your counseling suggestions (7). Thus, oral teaching, used exclusively, is not an effective technique (4).

Supplementing oral teaching with easy-to-read materials (words that are familiar and meaningful to clients) will improve clients' understanding and retention of information.

Additionally, the Latino client will often have family who can assist in the use and understanding of easy-to-read materials (7). Nutrition professionals need to learn to develop or select easy-to-read educational materials for all clients. It is also important to have easy-to-read materials (in appropriate Spanish) that you are comfortable using.

Personalization also aids understanding and is important to most clients. If possible, personalize printed materials by rewriting key points, by circling the applicable points, or by crossing out the parts that do not apply. Write in large, easy-to-read print (4). (See Section III for more information on health literacy.)

Behavior Change Models

Understanding motivation to change behavior is important for successful nutrition counseling. Many theories (models) have been proposed to explain how people make decisions to change behaviors. One theory (locus of control) applies to many Latinos; the stages of change (transtheoretical) model and the health belief model are summarized for comparison.

Stages of Change (Transtheoretical Model)

The Stages of Change model was developed by Prochaska and DiClemente in 1986 to understand smoking cessation behaviors (4). In this model, behavior change is explained as readiness to change. The stages are as follows:

- *Precontemplation:* the client is unaware or not interested in making the change.
- *Contemplation:* the client is thinking about making a change within the next six months.
- *Preparation:* the client decides to change and plans a change within the next month.
- *Action:* the client is trying to make the change and has been working at making the change for less than six months.
- *Maintenance:* the client works to sustain the change for six months or longer.

Specifically for nutrition counseling, difficulties arise when the intervention and the client's stage of change are mismatched (10).

Note that written materials and counseling styles are most often geared toward action, even though most clients are in the precontemplation or contemplation stages.

Health Belief Model

The Health Belief model was developed by the US Public Health Service in the 1950s to explain why people (especially those at high risk) did not participate in programs designed to detect or prevent disease. The Health Belief model shows us that clients are unlikely to take a health action unless they believe the following:

- Their health is in jeopardy.
- The disease would have serious effects, such as pain or loss of income.
- The benefits of taking action outweigh the costs of not taking action (and the action is within their grasp).
- There is a compelling "cue" for them to take action.

Cues to action include advice from respected sources (possibly a nutrition professional), media campaigns, or a friend's illness (4). Generally, a person's attitude toward their "nutrition lifestyle" is reflective of his or her attitude toward health (10).

Locus of Control

The Health Locus of Control theory (based on the Social Learning theory) is the degree to which individuals believe that their health is controlled by themselves or "powerful others." A client with an internal locus of control believes that health outcomes are directly the result of his or her behavior.

Most often a Latino client will have an external locus of control, believing that fate, luck, or chance is in control. Clients with an external locus of control are much more likely to hold the nutrition professional directly responsible for determining their action plan (4). In their book *Nutrition Counseling and Communication Skills*, Katharine Curry and Amy Jaffe describe the following way to promote behavior change for a client with an external locus of control without challenging the client's beliefs (10):

Client: *"My high blood sugar won't go away. I guess it is just my fate."*

Dietitian: *"Yes, I see. I have worked with some people with high blood sugar and it has been possible to control blood sugar fairly well. There is a nutrition plan that could have some effect on your blood sugar. Would you like to try it?"*

The importance of the family can also be used to motivate behavior change in Latino clients. For example, adults unwilling to make changes to benefit their own health may be motivated to change for the sake of their children (11).

References

1. Boyle M. *Community Nutrition in Action.* 3rd ed. Belmont, Calif: Wadsworth Publishing; 2003.

2. American Dietetic Association. *Ethnic and Regional Food Practices: Mexican-American.* 2nd ed. Chicago, Ill: American Dietetic Association; 1998.

3. Culture-sensitive health care: Hispanic. In: *From What Language Does Your Patient Hurt In? A Practical Guide to Culturally Competent Care.* Amherst, Mass: Diversity Resources; 2000. Available at: http://www.diversityresources.com/rc04_sample/hispanic.html. Accessed January 27, 2004.

4. Redman BK. *The Process of Patient Education.* 7th ed. St. Louis, Mo: Mosby Year Book; 1993.

5. Neuhouser ML, Thompson B, Coronado GD, Solomon CC. Higher fat intake and lower fruit and vegetables intake are associated with greater acculturation among Mexicans living in Washington state. *J Am Diet Assoc.* 2004;104:51-57.

6. Rodrigues JC. *Contemporary Nutrition for Latinos.* Lincoln, Neb: Universe, Inc; 2004.

7. Root J, Stableford S. *Write it Easy-to-Read: A Guide to Creating Plain English Materials.* Biddeford, Me: University of New England; 1998.

8. Clutter A. Understanding the Hispanic culture. Ohio State University fact sheet. HYG-5237-00. Available at: http://ohioline.osu.edu/hyg-fact/5000/5237.html. Accessed February 17, 2004.

9. Martinez RA. *Hispanic Culture and Health Care: Fact, Fiction, and Folklore.* St Louis, Mo: Mosby; 1978.

10. Curry K, Jaffe A. *Nutrition Counseling and Communication Skills.* Philadelphia, Pa: WB Saunders; 1998.

11. Kittler P, Sucher K. *Food and Culture in America.* 2nd ed. New York, NY: Van Nostrand Reinhold; 1997.

Spanish Grammar and Vocabulary for the Nutrition Professional

Chapter 7

Spanish Pronunciation

Vowels

Spanish is a very phonetic language and therefore is considered relatively easy to pronounce. Unlike English, the vowels in Spanish have only one sound regardless of where they appear in a Spanish word. The pronunciation of the Spanish vowels is as follows:

A Always pronounced "ah" as in the English word possible.
  Examples: *Ana, casa, papas, mar, cantar*

E A cross between the English "a" in words like cake or bake and the short English "e," as in bed.
  Examples: *mesa, rey, tres, Pepe, peso*

I Always pronounced like an English long "e" sound, as in beef or creek.
  Examples: *gris, piso, triste, privado, liso*

O Always pronounced like an English long "o" sound, as in home or broke.
  Examples: *como, rosa, sobre, sofá, Pedro*

U Always pronounced like the English long "u" sound, as in Bruce or food.
  Examples: *ruso, azul, Cuba, chulo, uvas*

Consonants

Although most consonants have the same or very similar sounds in English and Spanish, there are several consonants that have completely different sounds in Spanish. The differences are as follows:

C *(followed by e or i)* In Latin America and the United States, pronounced like the English "s."
  Examples: *cereza, cero, cine, centro*

C *(followed by a, o, or u and consonants)* In both Spain and

Latin America, pronounced like the English "k."
Examples: *cama, casa, coco, puerco, cuenta*

G *(followed by e or i)* Pronounced like the English "h."
Examples: *girafa, gente, giro, inteligente, Geraldo*

G *(followed by a, o, or u, or by a consonant)* Pronounced like the English "g" in guru, game, or go.
Examples: *gota, gato, goma, gusano, gris*

H Always silent in Spanish pronunciation.
Examples: *hola, hermano, Hugo, honesto, hogar*

J Always pronounced like the English "h," as in hunger or happy.
Examples: *José, Julia, juro, tejer, burbuja*

LL In most of Latin America and the United States, pronounced like the English consonant "y," as in yam.
Examples: *llama, llorar, Vallarta, llanto, amarillo*
In some parts of South America, "ll" can be pronounced like the English "j" in joke, or the English "sh" in shake. Those who pronounce "ll" this way will likely also pronounce the consonant "y" the same way.

Ñ Pronounced "ny" as in the English words onion or bunion.
Examples: *ñame, mañana, español, año, compañía*
Note: It is important to use the tilde (the curving line that appears above the "n") because this diacritical mark differentiates the pronunciation of "n" and "ñ." Some words in Spanish have identical pronunciation except for this letter but mean two completely different things, such as *campana* (bell), and *campaña* (campaign).

QU Pronounced like the English "k," as in kangaroo.
Examples: *quesadilla, tequila, queso, qué pasa, quiero*

R Always trilled when a word begins with "r." (English does not have this sound. Think of it as a slightly prolonged "r" sound.)
Examples: *Rodolfo, rojo, rico, roca, responsible*

R Always "tapped" within a word or at the end of a word. Similar to the "tt" sound in English words like butter, better, pitter, or patter.
Examples: *para, pero, hablar, caro, sudadera*

RR Always trilled in Spanish. (English does not have this sound. Think of it as a slightly prolonged "r" sound.)
Examples: *ferrocarril, perro, pizarra*

V In most of Latin America and the United States, the pronunciation of "v" is a combination of the English "v" and the English "b." For the nonnative speaker of Spanish, it will probably sound closer to the English "b."
Examples: *Valencia, Victor, veinte, vaca, vacaciones*
In some parts of Spain, "v" is pronounced as it is in English, as in victory.

Z In most of Latin America and the United States, pronounced like the English "s," as in Sara, syrup, or tacos.
Example: *Pizarra, zapato, Zócalo, zurdo, zorro*
In Spain, this consonant is pronounced like the English "th" in "thistle."

Depending on the region, there are other differences in pronunciation of consonants. For example, in parts of Puerto Rico and the Caribbean, "r" may be pronounced like "l" and vice versa (similar to the Chinese pronunciation of these consonants). However, most standard Spanish will be pronounced as explained above.

Spanish speakers, like English speakers, tend to blend syllables together, which gives the impression that Spanish is being spoken very rapidly. This will be frustrating at first, but by listening to native speakers of Spanish, you should eventually become accustomed to it. Try listening to a Spanish radio station or watching one of the Spanish television channels, such as Telemundo or Univsión, to get used to hearing Spanish.

Here's a Spanish tongue twister to practice with:
Pepe Pecas pica piedras con un pico. Con un pico Pepe Pecas pica piedras.

Accent Marks

There are three basic rules regarding which syllables receive stress in Spanish words. As with all rules, there are exceptions, which are detailed in most elementary Spanish texts. For our purposes, the three basic rules are as follows:

1. If a word ends in a vowel, an "n," or an "s," the stress will naturally fall on the penultimate (second to last) syllable of the word.
   Examples: ***Ho**/la, To/ci/**ni**/ta*
2. If a word ends in any other letter, the stress will naturally fall on the last syllable.
   Examples: *to/**mar**, na/**riz**, di/fi/cul/**tad***
3. If one of these two rules is broken, the word will carry a written accent mark to show that the accent is falling on a syllable that would normally be unstressed.
   Examples: ***lá**/piz, **rá**/pi/do*

Chapter 8

Adjectives in the Spanish Language

Gendered Adjectives

In the chapters that follow, many adjectives ending in the letter "o" can also be changed to end with the letter "a." In this book, these adjectives are noted with the ending o/a (for example, *descremado/a* [skim]). Which ending to use will depend on the gender of the noun that the adjective is describing. Nouns in Spanish are either masculine or feminine in gender, and when a noun of a certain gender is described with an adjective, that adjective should be in the same gender.

For example, *queso* (cheese) is a masculine noun, so if you refer to skim cheese, then you would use the masculine adjective *descremado* (ending in "o"). On the other hand, when speaking about skim milk, you would use the feminine version of the adjective because *leche* (milk) is a feminine noun.

Usually, but not always, masculine nouns will end in "o," and feminine nouns will end in "a." However, because there are nouns that end in other vowels or in consonants, it will not always be clear which form of the adjective should be used in describing the nouns. Although it won't be grammatically correct, when in doubt as to the gender of the noun, you may need to guess which form of the adjective to use.

Placement of Adjectives

In Spanish, adjectives are generally placed after nouns, unlike English, in which adjectives are placed before nouns. For example, "skim cheese" (adjective, noun) is translated as *queso descremado* (noun, adjective).

Plural Adjectives

If a noun is plural, then the adjective will be made plural too, by adding an "s" to the end. For example, "fresh apple" is translated *manzana fresca* whereas "fresh apples" is translated *manzanas frescas* (note that the Spanish word for "apples" is feminine).

You may want to refer to a Spanish grammar text, where these concepts will be explained in detail. Even if you are uncertain about the rules, don't be shy about trying to speak Spanish with your clients. In all but the rarest of cases, they will be happy that you are able to communicate in their language and will forgive your incorrect grammar.

Chapter 9

Introductory Conversation

This chapter presents some of the words and phrases you will need to have an introductory conversation with a Spanish-speaking person.

Ways to Greet Someone

Hello/Hi	*Hola*
Good morning	*Buenos días*
Good afternoon	*Buenas tardes*
Good evening	*Buenas noches*

After you've met someone, most Spanish-speaking people will shake hands and say:

Mucho gusto	Pleased to meet you
Encantada	Pleased to meet you (only said by females, to people of both genders)
Encantado	Pleased to meet you (only said by males, to people of both genders)

Cultural Tidbit

It is customary in Hispanic culture for two women, or one man and one woman, to greet each other with a kiss on one or both cheeks. This gesture is usually reserved for friends, but it is possible that someone you've just met may attempt to kiss your cheek. More likely, they may hug you. If a client greets you in this way, it may be considered rude for you not to reciprocate.

Introductory Questions and Answers

Question

How are you?	*¿Cómo está usted?*

Possible Responses

(Very) fine/well	*(Muy) bien*
So-so	*Así, así* or *Más o menos*
Not very well	*No muy bien*
(Very) bad	*(Muy) mal*

After being asked "*¿Cómo está usted?*" most people will answer the question, then say "*Gracias, ¿y usted?*" (Thank you, and you?).

Question

What is your name?	*¿Cómo se llama usted?* or *¿Cuál es su nombre?*

Response

My name is _____.	*Me llamo_____.*

Question

What country are you from?	*¿De qué país es usted?*

Response

I am from_____.	*(Yo) soy de_____.*

Titles in Spanish

Titles that are used in Spanish include the following:

Mrs.	*Señora*
Miss/Ms.	*Señorita*
Mr.	*Señor*

It is a common sign of respect to use the above titles, even without surnames attached, when greeting someone. For example, *Hola, Señora,* or *Hola, Señor. ¿Cómo está usted?*

The titles *Don* and *Doña* are used before first names with older friends, neighbors, or godparents. You probably will not want to use these titles with clients, at least until you are better acquainted with them.

Cultural Tidbit

Personal space for Latinos tends to be closer than that of non-Latino Americans. In general, Latinos may touch each other more than non-Latino Americans.

Ways to Say Good-bye

The following are some of the words and phrases you might use before leaving a client:

Good-bye	*Adiós*
See you later	*Hasta luego* or *Hasta la vista*
See you tomorrow	*Hasta mañana*
See you soon	*Hasta pronto*
We'll see each other	*Nos vemos*

You should practice these words and phrases as often as possible until they become second nature. Any Spanish-speaking person you encounter will probably be very happy to have a miniconversation with you. But beware: if you begin speaking Spanish with a native speaker, he or she might want to continue the conversation, speaking very rapidly and saying things you don't understand. What do you say?

"Lo siento, pero hablo muy poco español." (I'm sorry, but I speak very little Spanish.)

Or, if you already know some Spanish but are finding it difficult to follow the conversation, you can say:

"¿Podría hablar más despacio, por favor?" (Could you please speak more slowly?)

Chapter 10

Numbers from 1 to 1,000

From 0 to 15

Numbers in Spanish follow a series of patterns, just as they do in English. The first group of numbers, which must be memorized, is from 0 to 15.

0	*cero*
1	*uno*
2	*dos*
3	*tres*
4	*cuatro*
5	*cinco*
6	*seis*
7	*siete*
8	*ocho*
9	*nueve*
10	*diez*
11	*once*
12	*doce*
13	*trece*
14	*catorce*
15	*quince*

From 16 to 99

Beginning with 16, Spanish numbers follow a pattern whereby the number spoken in the tens place indicates the number of tens, followed by *y* (the word for "and"), then the number of ones.

For example:

16	*diez y seis* (ten and six) (also written as *dieciséis*)
17	*diez y siete* (ten and seven) (also written as *diecisiete*)
18	*diez y ocho* (ten and eight) (also written as *dieciocho*)
19	*diez y nueve* (ten and nine) (also written as *diecinueve*)

Note: The one-word spelling is much more common, but the three-word spelling is a bit easier to remember. Just remember to pronounce the three words as one.

Because all Spanish numbers from 16 to 99 follow this same pattern, it is only necessary to memorize the numbers for 20, 30, 40, 50, 60, 70, 80, and 90.

20	*veinte*
30	*treinta*
40	*cuarenta*
50	*cincuenta*
60	*sesenta*
70	*setenta*
80	*ochenta*
90	*noventa*

When you want to express a number within these units of ten, simply add *y* and then the number from 1 to 9. For example:

66	*sesenta y seis*
43	*cuarenta y tres*
79	*setenta y nueve*

These numbers are usually pronounced rapidly, more like a single word instead of three separate words.

From 100 to 1,000

The numbers from 100 to 1,000 in Spanish are as follows:

100	*cien* (Note: *Cien* is used when the number counted is exactly 100. *Ciento* is used when another number follows *cien*—for example, *ciento uno* [101]).
200	*doscientos*
300	*trescientos*
400	*cuatrocientos*
500	*quinientos*
600	*seiscientos*
700	*setecientos*
800	*ochocientos*
900	*novecientos*
1,000	*mil* (Tip: think "millennium")

When counting objects that are assigned a feminine gender in Spanish, the adjective *cienta* is used instead of *ciento*, and the numbers 200 through 900 end with "as" instead of "os"—for example, *doscientas* or *trescientas*. For more information on the concept of gender agreement in Spanish grammar, see Chapter 8.

When counting numbers from 100 to 999, no *y* is needed between the number in the hundreds and the number being added to it. For example:

356	*trescientos cincuenta y seis* (not *trescientos y cincuenta y seis*)

The *y* is also not used when stating numbers in the thousands. For example:

25,589	*veinticinco mil, quinientos ochenta y nueve*

Cultural Tidbit

When writing numbers, people in some Spanish-speaking countries use periods where people in the United States use commas, and vice versa. For example, what is written as 25,589 in the United States is written 25.589 in some Spanish-speaking countries. It is important to discover which system of punctuation a client uses to avoid miscommunication.

The best way to learn Spanish numbers is to practice counting. Try to get in the habit of counting in Spanish in the shower, at a stoplight, or when doing your sit-ups. Any time you would normally count in English, count in Spanish instead.

Chapter 11

Telling Time

Discussing Time with Your Client

When interacting with clients, you will not be asking them what time it is, but rather, at what time they did something. The question "at what time?" is expressed *"¿A qué hora?"* It is answered using one of the following two formulas:

A __la__ + the time of day for any time between 1:00 and 1:59.

A __las__ + time of day for any time between 2:00 and 12:59.

For example:

Question

At what time?   *¿A qué hora?*

Responses

At 1:00.   *A la una.*

At 2:00.   *A las dos.*

At 3:00.   *A las tres.*

When the time is not exactly on the hour, in Spanish, as in English, the minutes are simply added to the hour, using the conjunction *y* (and) or the preposition *con* (with).

For example:

Question

At what time?   *¿A qué hora?*

Responses

At 1:12.   *A la una y doce.* or
                                 A la una con doce.

At 9:20.   *A las nueve y veinte.* or
                                 A las nueve con veinte.

When the time is "quarter past" or "half past" the hour, the following phrases are often used:

| quarter after | *y cuarto* |
| half past | *y media* |

For example:

Question

| At what time? | *¿A qué hora?* |

Responses

| At 5:15. | *A las cinco y cuarto.* |
| At 10:30. | *A las diez y media.* |

Although *y cuarto* and *y media* are more often used to express "quarter after" and "half past," it is also acceptable to use the numbers *quince* and *treinta*.

When the time is more than half past the hour (between 31 minutes and 59 minutes past the hour), there are two ways to express this in Spanish. The simplest way is to simply add the minutes to the hour, as in the examples above.

For example:

| At 1:55. | *A la una y cincuenta y cinco.* |
| At 12:45. | *A las doce y cuarenta y cinco.* |

The second way to express this is to count up to the next hour, and then subtract the minutes left until that hour strikes, using the word *menos*. For example, 1:55 could be expressed as *A la una y cincuenta y cinco* or as *A las dos menos cinco*. The latter way is more commonly used. However, it may be easier for you to simply add the minutes to the hour.

A.M. or P.M.?

There are two ways to express the English phrases "in the morning," "in the afternoon," or "at night," depending on whether the phrases are attached to a specific hour.

Specific Hour

When using these phrases in conjunction with a specific hour, Spanish uses:

in the morning	*de la mañana*
in the afternoon	*de la tarde*
at night	*de la noche*

For example:

At 8:00 in the morning.	*A las ocho de la mañana.*
At 3:30 in the afternoon.	*A las tres y media de la tarde.*
At 7:45 at night.	*A las ocho menos cuarto de la noche.*

General Time of Day

When speaking of morning, afternoon, or evening as general times of day, Spanish uses:

in the morning	*por la mañana* or *en la mañana*
in the afternoon	*por la tarde* or *en la tarde*
at night	*por la noche* or *en la noche*

Military Time

Some Spanish speakers may be accustomed to using military time because this is the practice in some countries. In military time, the hours of the day are counted from 0 (midnight) to 23 (11:00 p.m.)—1:00 p.m. is 1300, 2:00 p.m. is 1400, and so on. For example, "at 1615" (4:15 p.m.) translates as *a las dieciséis y cuarto*.

Chapter 12

What Do You Eat?
When Do You Eat?

Eating Habits

Individuals in Spanish-speaking countries generally enjoy three meals a day and occasional snacks, much like individuals in the United States. Of course, the content of those meals will vary greatly, as will the size of the meals and the time of day they are eaten.

In the United States, dinner is generally considered the main meal of the day and is consumed in the early to mid-evening. In contrast, individuals in most Spanish-speaking countries consider lunch their main meal, and dinner is usually lighter and eaten later. Many stores and businesses in these countries close down for a few hours mid-day so that all family members can enjoy their main meal together, although this practice is not as prevalent as it once was, especially in larger cities. Children generally come home from school to have lunch. Sometimes people take a *siesta*, a short afternoon nap, after lunch.

Breakfast in Spanish-speaking countries tends to be lighter than a traditional American breakfast. Breakfast consists of strong coffee, juices, fresh fruits, sweet breads, and pastries. Sometimes eggs and a breakfast meat may be served. Beans are also a staple breakfast food in many Spanish-speaking countries. Breakfast in Spanish-speaking countries is usually eaten at about the same time (early to mid-morning) as in the United States.

In Spanish-speaking countries, a snack is usually eaten between lunch and dinner, at around 5:00 or 6:00 p.m. Snacks often consist of sweet bread, pastries, *churros*, cookies, and hot drinks, such as coffee or hot chocolate.

It is very important to note here that these are general characteristics of Latino mealtimes and eating habits. Just as there are many different Spanish-speaking countries and cultures, there is also great variety in the foods that are consumed.

Names of Meals

The names of the meals in Spanish-speaking countries are:

breakfast	*desayuno*
lunch	*almuerzo*
	also used: *comida; lonche*

[**Note:** Sometimes the terms *desayuno* and *almuerzo* are used interchangeably.]

dinner	*cena*
snack	*merienda*
	also used: *bocadillo; entrecomidas*

Desayuno (breakfast) is normally eaten *por la mañana* (in the morning); *almuerzo, comida,* or *lonche* (lunch) is generally eaten *por la tarde* (in the afternoon); and *cena* (dinner) is eaten *por la noche* (at night).

Common Adverbs

Some adverbs used when talking about meals are:

always	*siempre*
generally	*generalmente*
never	*nunca*
normally	*normalmente*
usually	*usualmente*

Basic Questions and Answers

Some questions and phrases relating to meals are:

Do you eat . . . ?	*¿Come usted . . . ?*
When?	*¿Cúando?*
I eat . . .	*(Yo) como . . .* *
I don't eat . . .	*(Yo) no como . . .* *
Are you hungry?	*¿Tiene usted hambre?*
Are you thirsty?	*¿Tiene usted sed?*
I am hungry.	*(Yo) tengo hambre.* *

I am thirsty.   *(Yo) tengo sed.**

Yo (I) is optional.

Practice Dialogues

These questions and answers can be combined with the questions and phrases you've already learned to form dialogues. Read the following dialogue between a nutrition professional (*nutricionista*) and a client (*cliente*):

Nutricionista: *Señora Mendoza, ¿cuándo come usted el desayuno?* (Mrs. Mendoza, when do you eat breakfast?)

Cliente: *Como el desayuno por la mañana.* (I eat breakfast in the morning.)

Nutricionista: *¿A qué hora come usted el desayuno?* (What time do you eat breakfast?)

Cliente: *Normalmente como el desayuno a las ocho de la mañana.* (Usually I eat breakfast at 8:00 a.m.)

Nutricionista: *¿Y a qué hora come usted el almuerzo y la cena, normalmente?* (And what time do you usually eat lunch?)

Cliente: *Generalmente como el almuerzo a las doce y media, y la cena a las siete.* (I generally eat lunch at 12:30, and dinner at 7:00.)

Nutricionista: *¿Come usted una merienda?* (Do you eat a snack?)

Cliente: *Sí, como una merienda a las cuatro y media, más o menos.* (Yes, I eat a snack at around 4:30.)

After practicing this dialogue a few times, try to write your own dialogue. The dialogue can be lengthened by adding some of the basic conversation vocabulary you previously learned. Find a partner to help you practice each of the dialogues you've created. Then try having an impromptu conversation.

Chapter 13

Breakfast Foods

artificial sweetener	*endulzante (artificial)*
avacado	*aguacate*
bacon*	*tocino*
	also used: *tocineta; panceta*
beans (dried)	*frijoles*
	also used: *habichuelas;*
	porotos
bread (see also: toast)	*pan* (for image, see
	Chapter 15)
wheat bread	*pan de trigo*
white bread	*pan blanco*
whole-grain bread	*pan integral*
bread roll	*bolillo; panecillo*
butter	*mantequilla*
	also used: *manteca*
	(however, this word often
	refers to lard)
cereal*	*cereal*
	also used: *maizoro*
cheese*	*queso*
coffee*	*café*
coffee with milk	*café con leche*
cream	*crema*
	also used: *nata*

*Chapter includes an image of this food.

eggs*	*huevos* (Caution: Some cultures consider this word obscene. However, a majority of Spanish-speaking individuals equate this term with eggs.) also used: *blanquillos*
egg white	*clara de huevo* also used: *clara de blanquillo*
egg yolk	*yema de huevo* also used: *yema de blanquillo*
french toast	*torrija* also used: *torreja*
fruits*	*frutas*
ham*	*jamón*
hash browns	*papas doradas*
honey	*miel de abeja*
jelly*	*jalea* also used: *mermelada; dulce*
juice	*jugo* also used: *zumo*
apple juice	*jugo de manzana*
cranberry juice	*jugo de arándano*
grape juice	*jugo de uva*
orange juice	*jugo de naranja* also used: *jugo de china*
tomato juice	*jugo de tomate* also used: *jugo de jitomate*
margarine	*margarina*
milk*	*leche*
chocolate milk	*leche de chocolate*
evaporated milk	*leche evaporada*
sweetened condensed milk	*leche condensada*

*Chapter includes an image of this food.

oatmeal*	*avena*
pancakes*	*panqueques* also used: *panques; crepas;* *panquecas; hotcakes*
pastry*	*pan dulce*
plantain	*plátano* also used: *plátano macho;* *plátano grande*
sausage*	*salchicha* also used: *chorizo*
sugar	*azúcar*
syrup	*almíbar* also used: *sirope*
tea	*té*
toast*	*pan tostado*
wheat toast	*pan de trigo tostado*
white toast	*pan blanco tostado*
whole-grain toast	*pan integral tostado*
tortilla	*tortilla*
corn tortilla	*tortilla de maiz*
flour tortilla	*tortilla de harina*
waffles	*wafles*
yogurt	*yogur* (for image, see Chapter 14)

Chapter includes an image of this food.

bacon

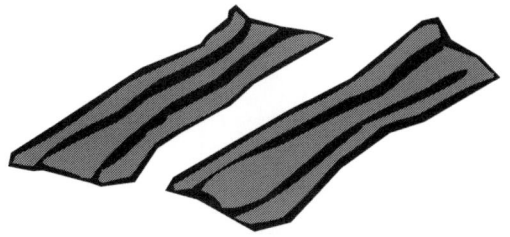

tocino
also used: *tocineta; panceta*

cereal

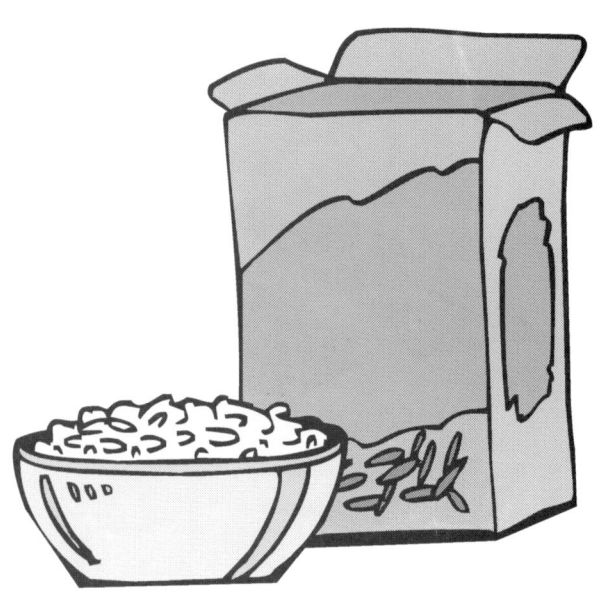

cereal

cheese

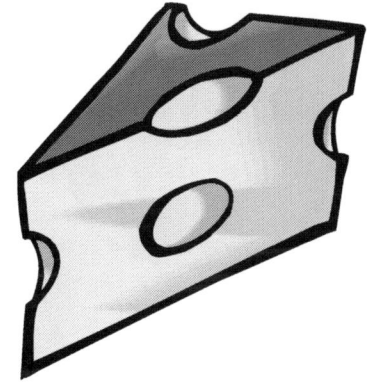

queso

coffee

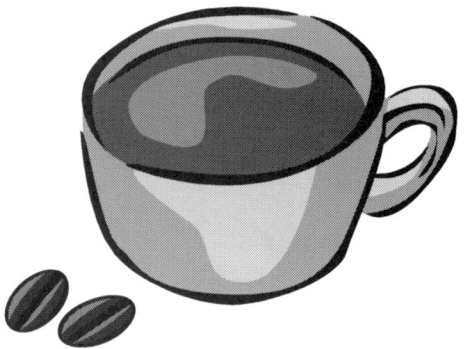

café

eggs

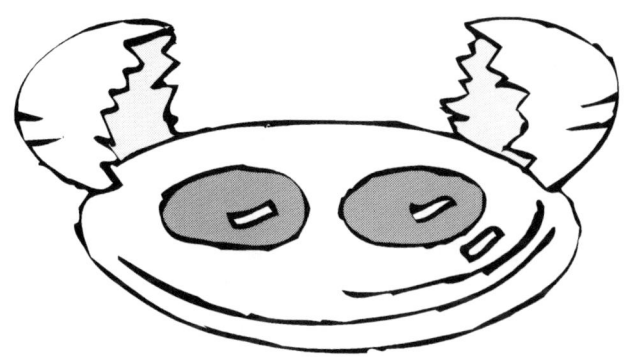

huevos
also used: *blanquillos*

fruits

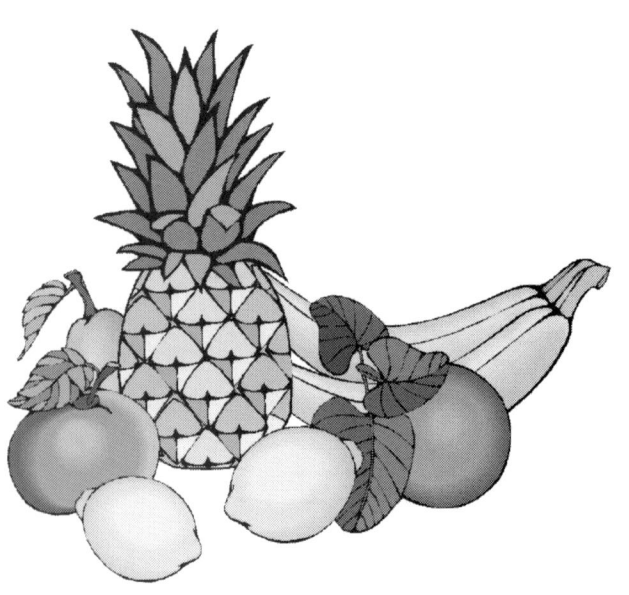

frutas

ham

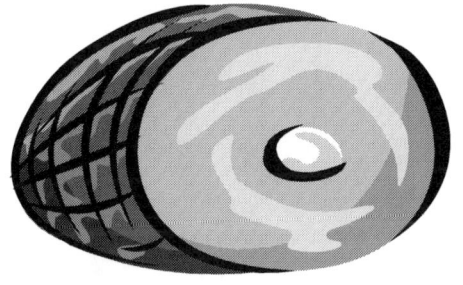

jamón

jelly

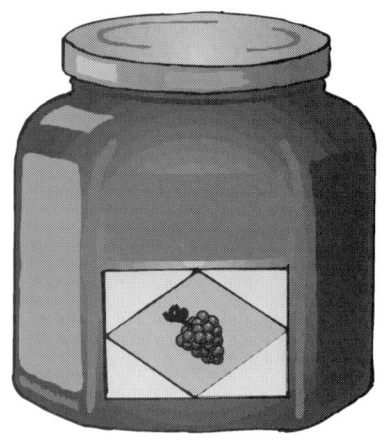

jalea
also used: *mermelada; dulce*

milk

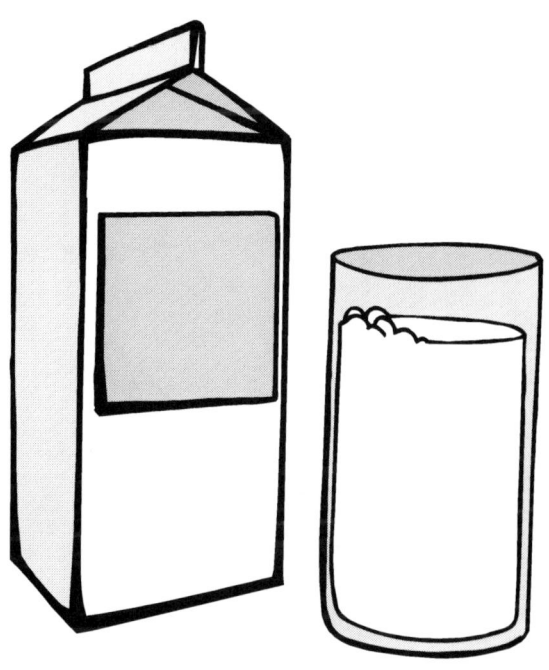

leche

oatmeal

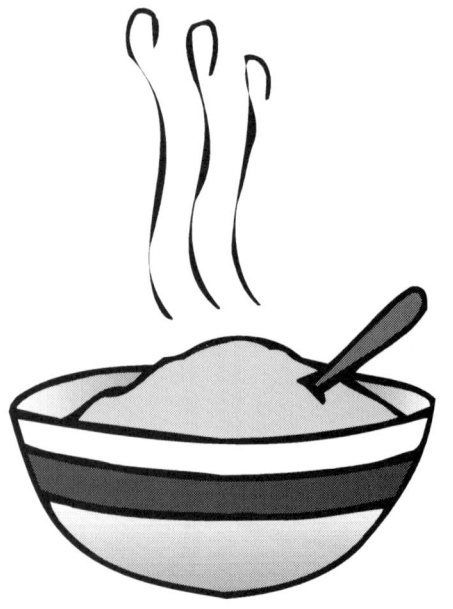

avena

pancakes

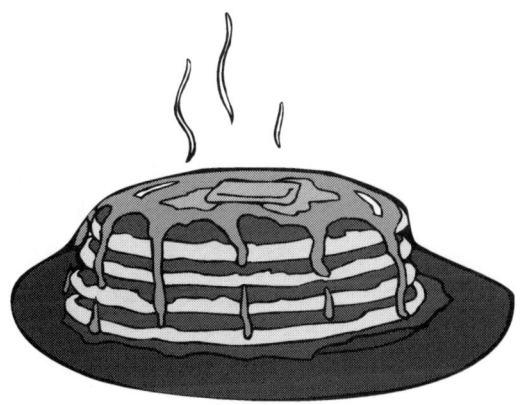

panqueques
also used: *panques; crepas; panquecas; hotcakes*

pastry

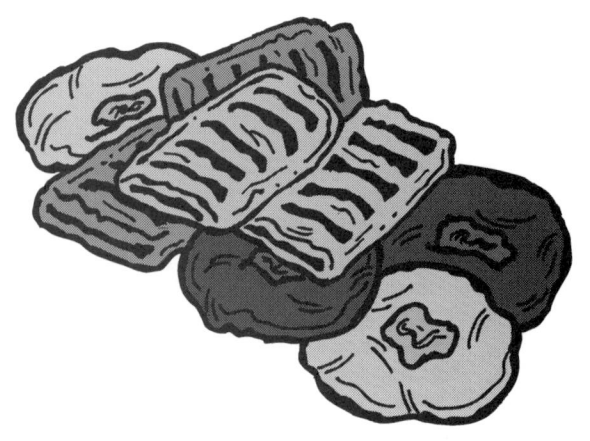

pan dulce

sausage

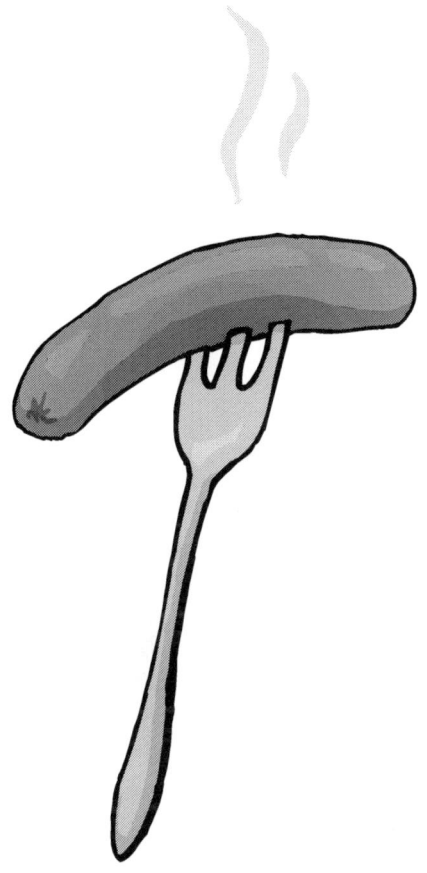

salchicha
also used: *chorizo*

toast

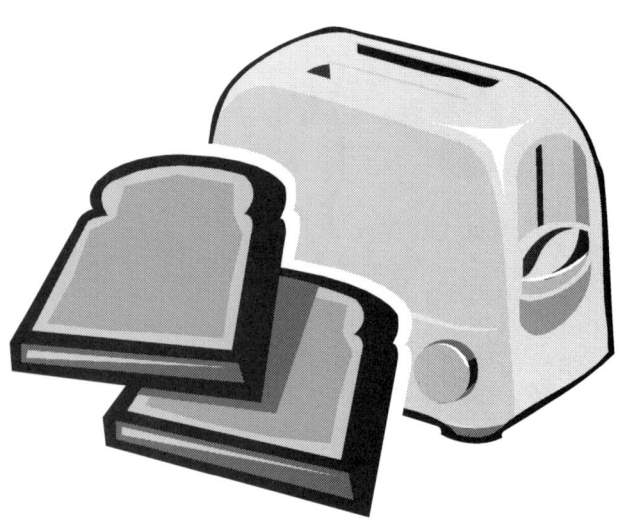

pan tostado

Chapter 14

Lunch Foods

Note: Many of the foods listed in this section are also eaten for dinner.

chips (snack)	*chips* also used: *totopos; papitas de bolsa; papitas fritas; tostaditas*
cold cuts	*carne para sándwich*
cole slaw	*ensalada de col* also used: *ensalada de repollo*
french fries*	*papas fritas* also used: *papitas*
fried pork skins	*chicharrones*
grilled cheese sandwich	*sándwich de queso fundido*
hamburger*	*hamburguesa*
hot dog*	*hot dog* also used: *pancho; salchica*
ketchup	*catsup* also used: *salsa de tomate; salsa de jitomate* (these terms are also used for tomato sauce)
mayonnaise	*mayonesa*
mustard	*mostaza*
peanut butter*	*crema de cacahuate* also used: *crema de maní; mantequilla de cacahuate; mantequilla de maní*

*Chapter includes an image of this food.

pizza*	*pizza*
pretzel*	*prétzel*
saltines/crackers	*galletas saladas*
sandwich*	*sándwich* also used: *torta; bocadillo* (*bocadillo* may also refer to a snack or appetizer); *emparedado*
[type of] sandwich	*sándwich de* [type]
smoothie	*licuado* (Note: A *licuado* is a pureed fruit drink with water, ice, and sugar, sometimes with milk and a raw egg. To describe the type of smooth- ie, one would say "*licuado de . . .* "—for example, *licuado de fresa* [strawberry smoothie] or *licuado de piña* [pineapple smoothie].)
soft drink*	*refresco* also used: *gaseosa; soda*
diet soft drink	*refresco dieta* also used: *gaseosa dieta; refresco lite; gaseosa lite*
spaghetti*	*espaguetis* also used: *espaguettis*
water	*agua*
yogurt*	*yogur*

Chapter includes an image of this food.

french fries

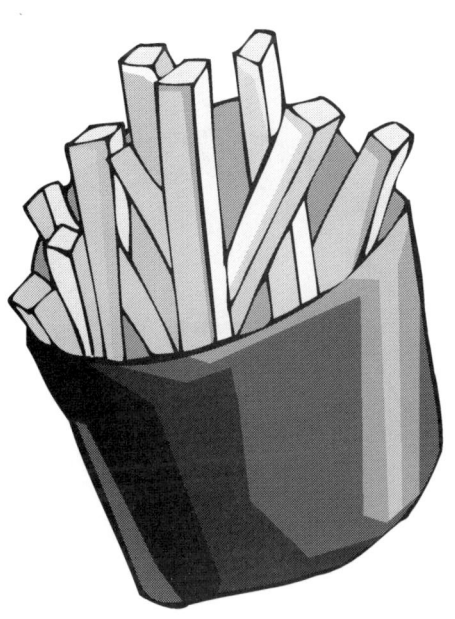

papas fritas
also used: *papitas*

hamburger

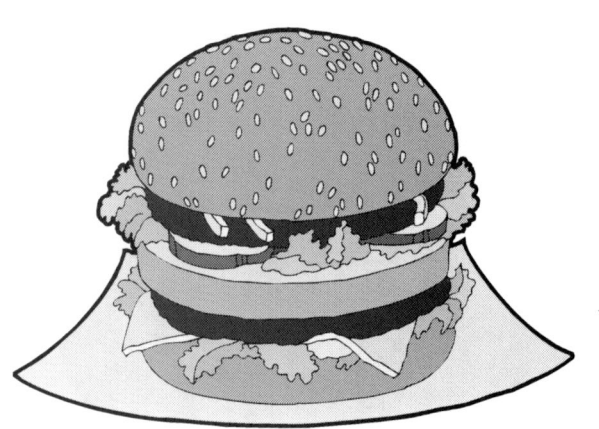

hamburguesa

hot dog

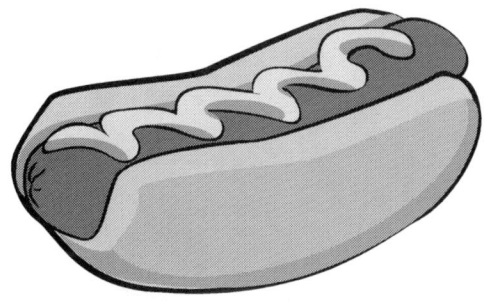

hot dog
also used: *pancho; salchica*

peanut butter

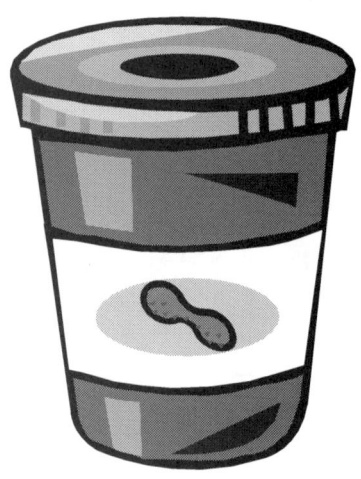

crema de cacahuate
also used: *crema de maní; mantequilla de cachuate; mantequilla de maní*

pizza

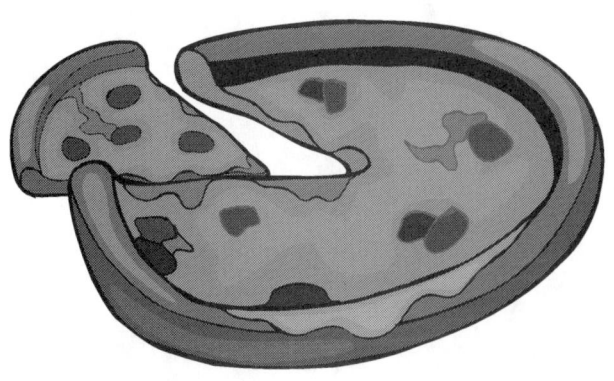

pizza

pretzel

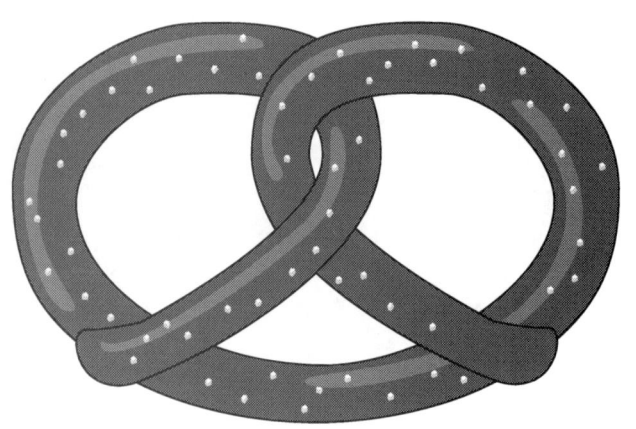

prétzel

sandwich

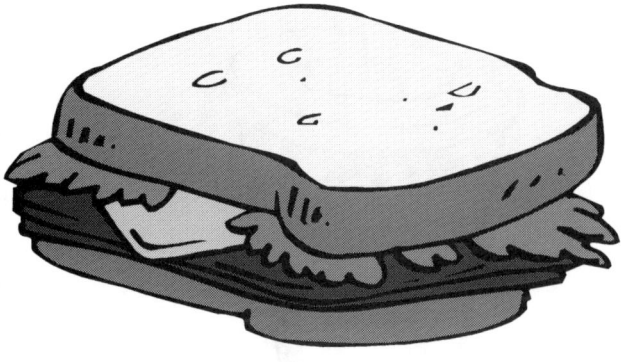

sándwich
also used: *torta; bocadillo; emparedado*

soft drink

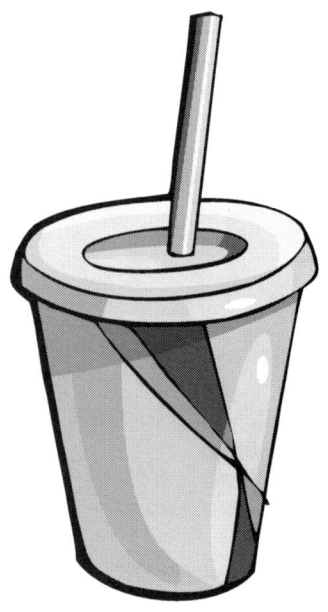

refresco
also used: *gaseosa; soda*

spaghetti

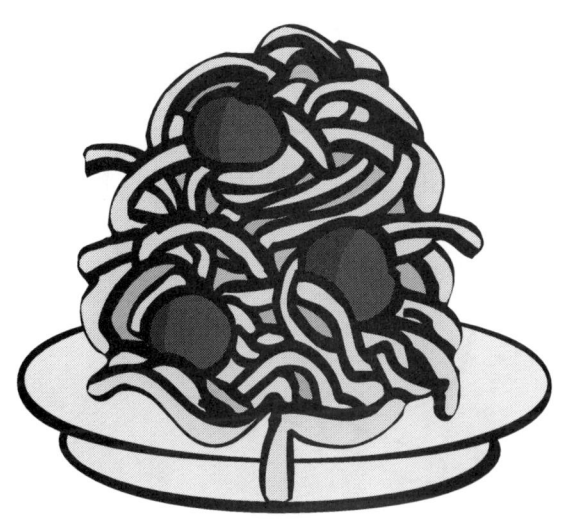

espaguetis
also used: *espaguettis*

yogurt

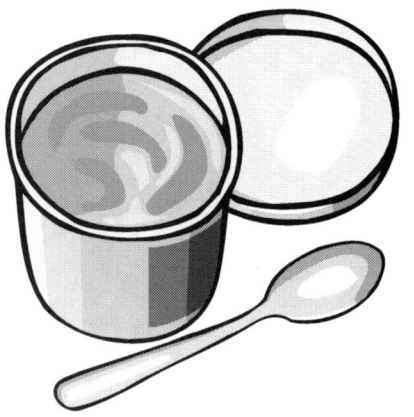

yogur

Chapter 15

Dinner Foods

Note: Many of these foods are also eaten for lunch.

beef	*carne de res* also used: *carne roja*
ground beef	*carne molida* also used: *carne picada*
bread*	*pan*
cheese	*queso*
chicken*	*pollo*
fish*	*pescado*
shellfish*	*mariscos*
tuna	*atún*
ham	*jamón*
liver	*hígado*
noodles*	*fideos*
pork chop*	*chuleta de puerco* also used: *chuleta de cerdo;* *costillo de cerolo*
rice*	*arroz*
salad*	*ensalada*
salad dressing	*aderezo* also used: *aliño, condimento*
soup*	*sopa* (Note: In northern Mexico, *sopa* may also refer to a dish with pasta and tomatoes.)
spaghetti	*espaguetis* (for image, see Chapter 14) also used: *espaguettis*

*Chapter includes an image of this food.

steak*	*bistec* also used: *bife*
turkey*	*pavo* also used: *guajolote* (Note: some people use *guajolote* to refer only to a live turkey.)

*Chapter includes an image of this food.

bread

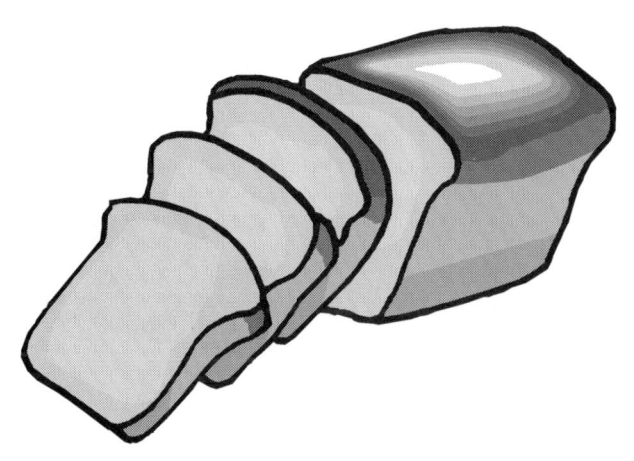

pan

chicken

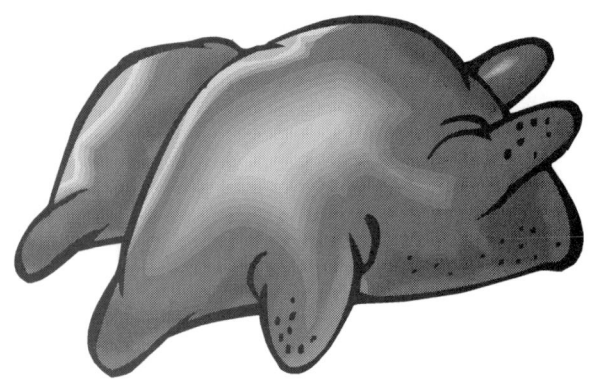

pollo

fish

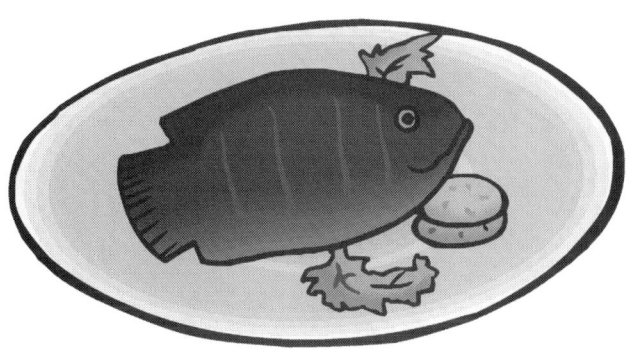

pescado

noodles

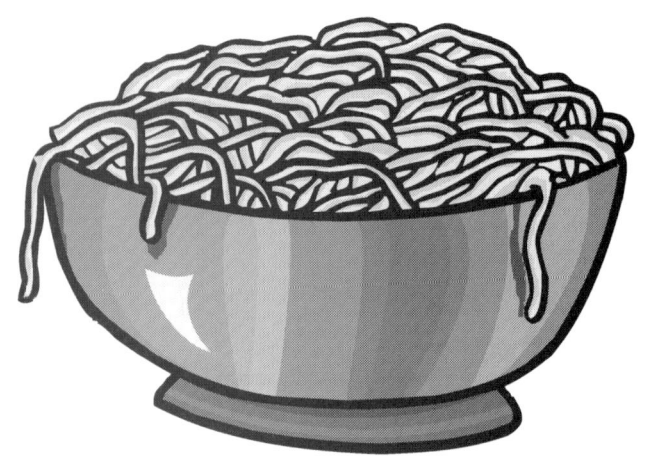

fideos

pork chop

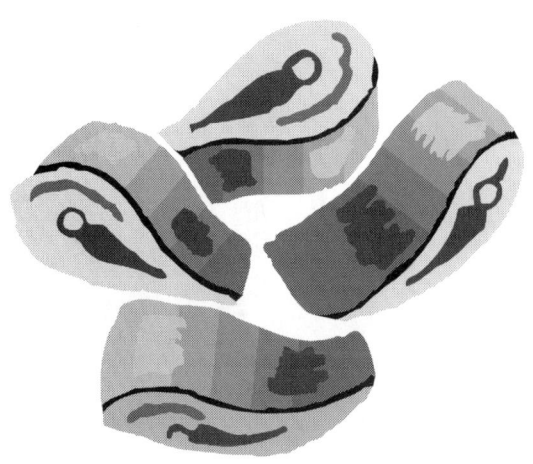

chuleta de puerco
also used: *chuleta de cerdo; costillo de cerolo*

rice

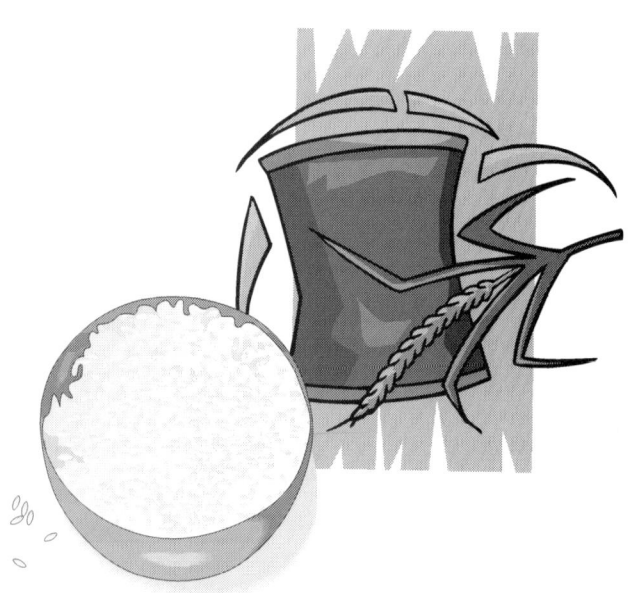

arroz

salad

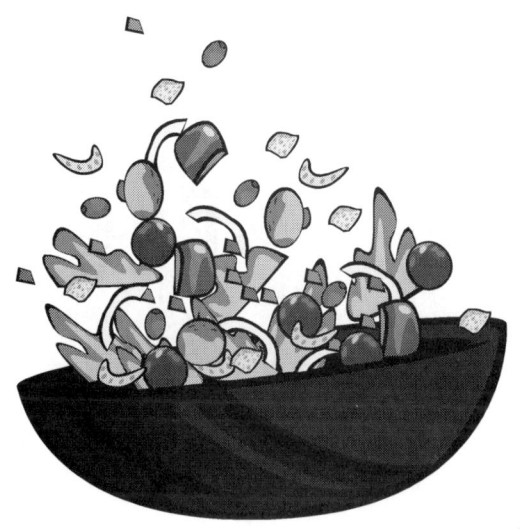

ensalada

shellfish

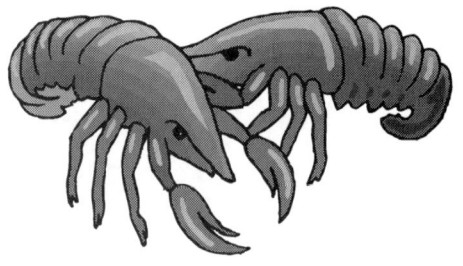

mariscos

soup

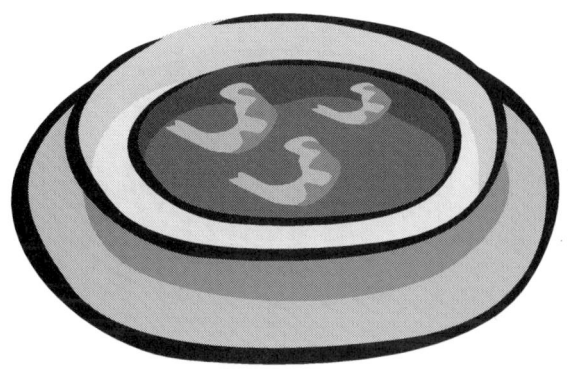

sopa

steak

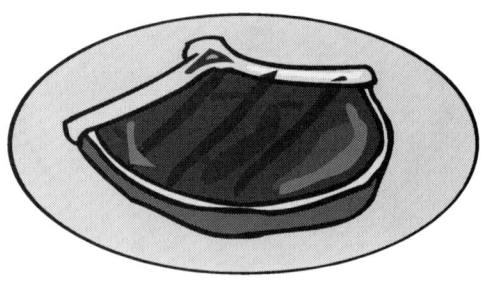

bistec
also used: *bife*

turkey

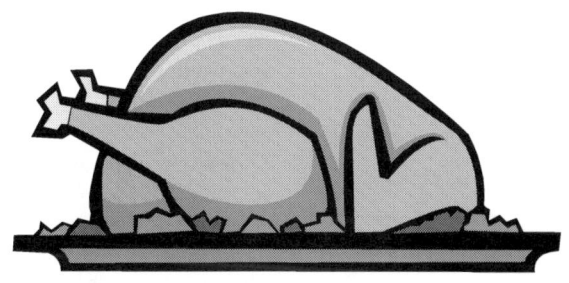

pavo
also used: *guajolote*

Chapter 16

Desserts and Sweets

cake*	*pastel* also used: *torta; biscocho* (Caution: *Biscocho* is the word most commonly used for "cake" in the Caribbean. In Mexico, this term is often considered obscene.]
candy; sweets*	*dulces* also used: *caramelos;* *golosinas*
chocolate or hot chocolate	*chocolate* To describe a chocolate-fla- vored food: [type of food] *de* *chocolate*. For example, *pastel de chocolate* trans- lates as "chocolate cake."
cookies*	*galletas dulces*
cupcake*	*pastelito* also used: *magdalena;* *cubilete; mantecada;* *pastelillo*
custard	*flan*
donuts*	*donas* also used: *rosquillas*
gelatin	*gelatina*
ice cream*	*helado* also used: *nieve*

Chapter includes an image of this food.

muffin*	*panque* also used: *panecillo; mollete; muffin*
pie*	*pai* also used: *pastel; empana- da; tarta; torta*
pudding	*pudin*
sherbet/sorbet	*sorbete* or *helado de nieve* also used: *helado de agua*
sweets	*dulces*

*Chapter includes an image of this food.

cake

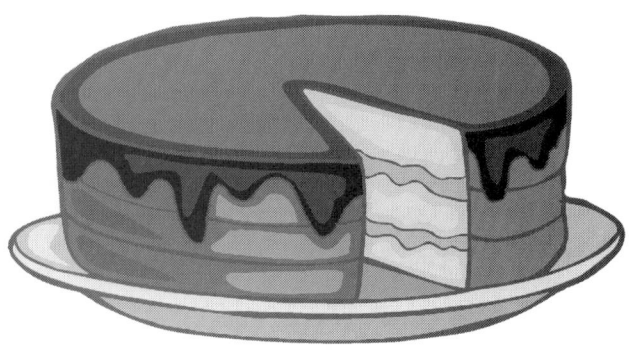

pastel

also used: *torta; biscocho*

candy; sweets

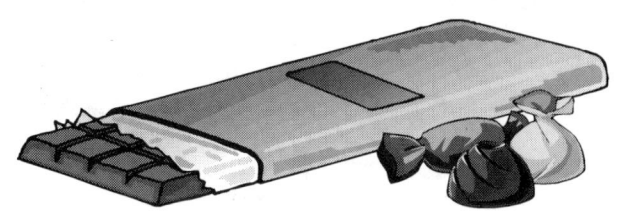

dulces
also used: *caramelos; golosinas*

cookies

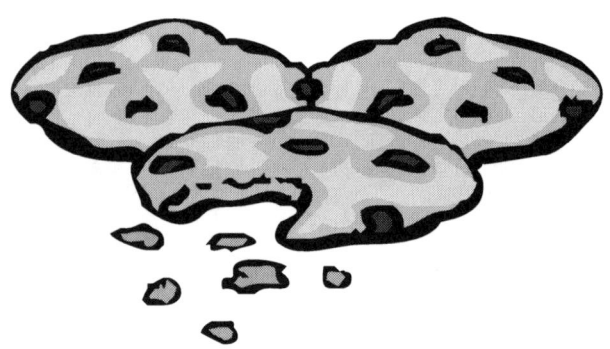

galletas dulces

cupcake

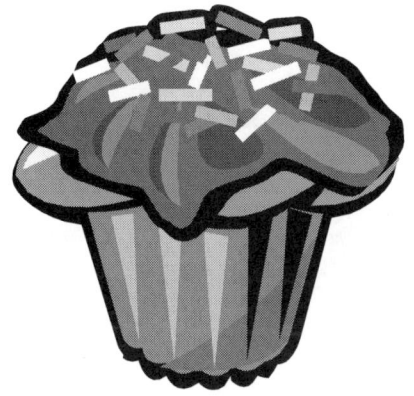

pastelito
**also used: *magdalena; cubilete;
mantecada; pastelillo***

donuts

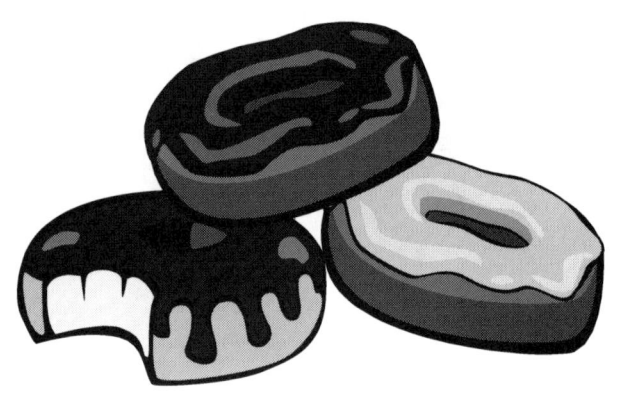

donas
also used: *rosquillas*

ice cream

helado
also used: *nieve*

muffin

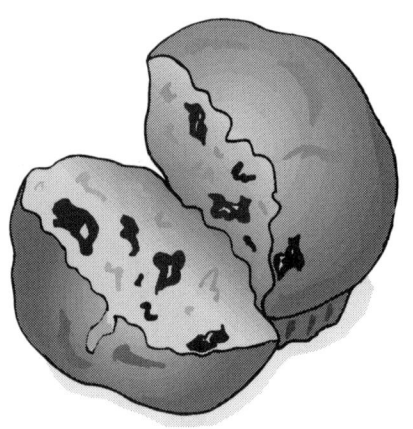

panque
also used: *panecillo; mollete; muffin*

pie

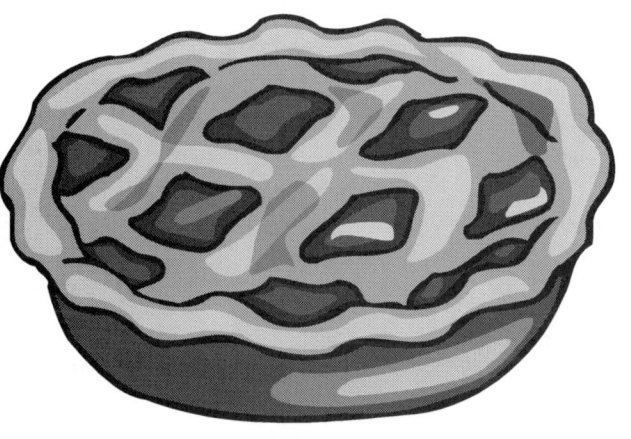

pai
also used: *pastel; empanada; tarta; torta*

Chapter 17

Vegetables

broccoli*	*brócoli*
	also used: *brécol*
brussels sprouts	*col de Bruselas*
	also used: *Bruselas;*
	repollitos de Bruselas;
	colecitas de Bruselas
cabbage	*col*
	also used: *repollo*
cactus*	*nopal*
	also used: *nopalitos*
carrot*	*zanahoria*
cauliflower*	*coliflor*
corn	*maíz*
corn on the cob*	*elote*
	also used: *mazorca de maíz;*
	choclo de maíz
cucumber*	*pepino*
dark-green leafy vegetables	*verduras de hojas verdes*
green beans*	*judías verdes*
	also used: *ejotes; porotos*
	verdes; habichuelas
green bell pepper*	*pimiento verde*
	also used: *chile verde; aji*
	verde; chile ancho
green peas*	*guisantes*
	also used: *chícharos; petit*
	pois (pronounced *petipuás*);
	arvejas

Chapter includes an image of this food.

jicama	*jicama*
lettuce*	*lechuga*
onion*	*cebolla*
potatoes*	*papas* also used: *patatas*
pumpkin*	*calabaza*
spinach*	*espinacas* also used: *espinaca*
sweet potatoes	*batatas* also used: *camotes;* *boniatos*
tomato*	*tomate* also used: *jitomate*
zucchini*	*calabacita* also used: *calabacín;* *zapallito*

Chapter includes an image of this food.

broccoli

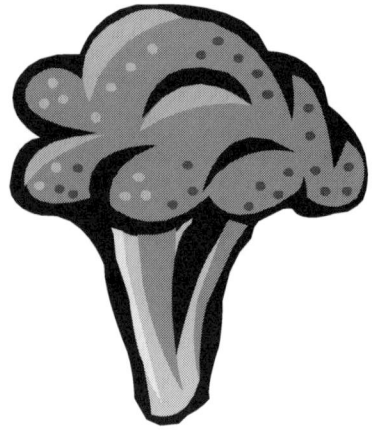

brócoli
also used: *brécol*

cactus

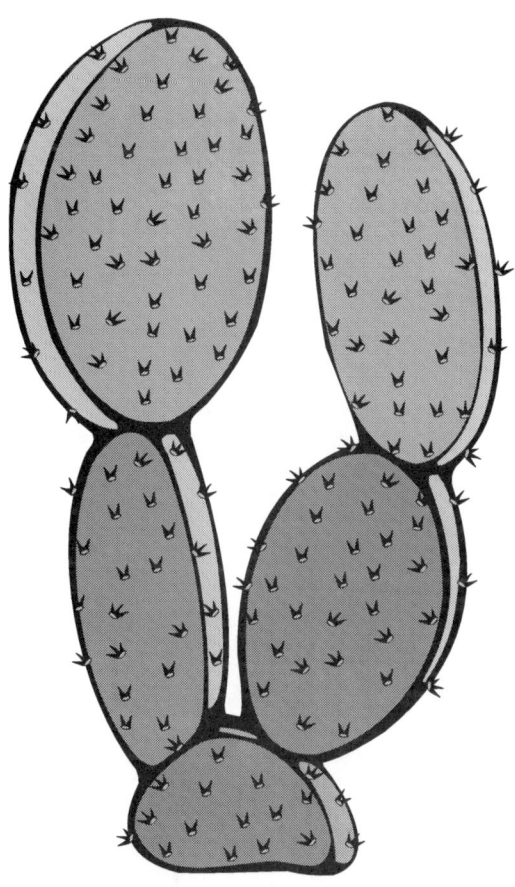

nopal
also used: *nopalitos*

carrot

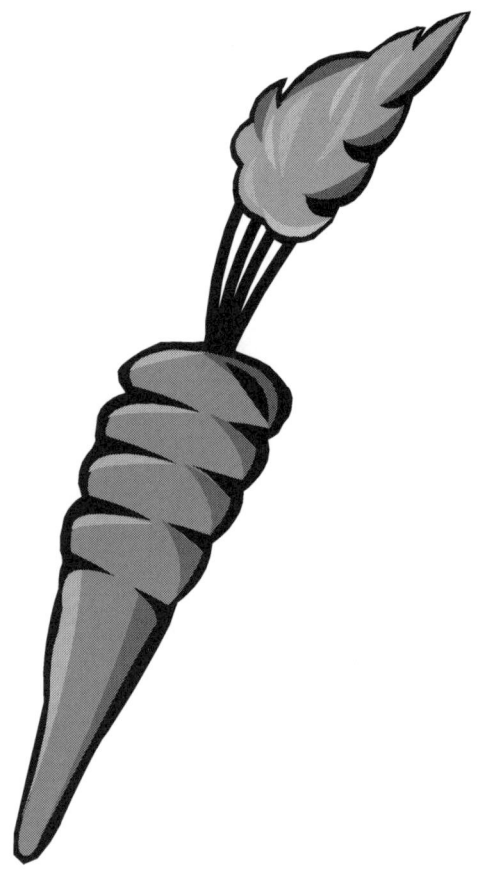

zanahoria

cauliflower

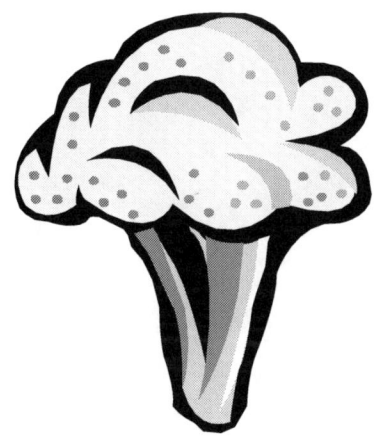

coliflor

corn on the cob

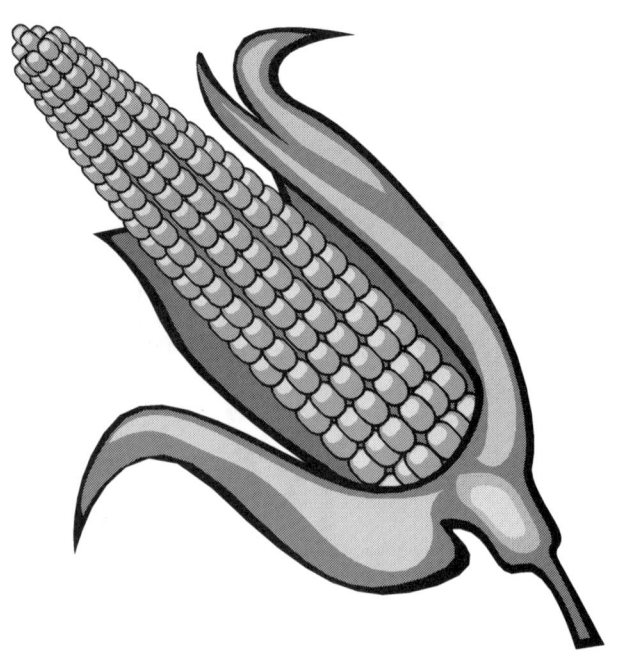

elote
also used: *mazorca de maíz;*
choclo de maíz

cucumber

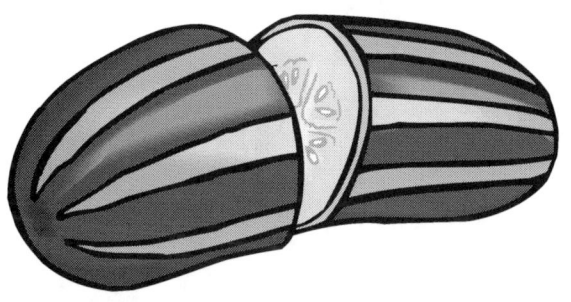

pepino

green beans

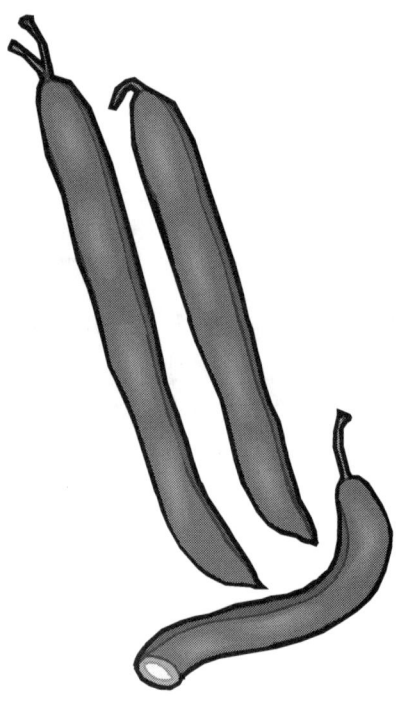

judías verdes
**also used: ejotes; porotos verdes;
habichuelas**

green bell pepper

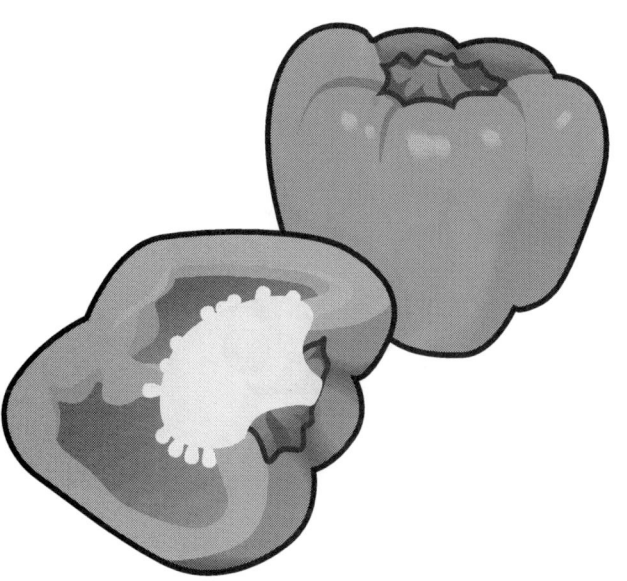

pimiento verde
also used: *chile verde; aji verde; chile ancho*

green peas

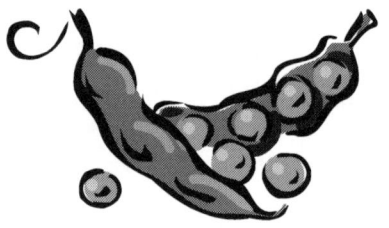

guisantes
also used: *chícaros; petit pois; arvejas*

lettuce

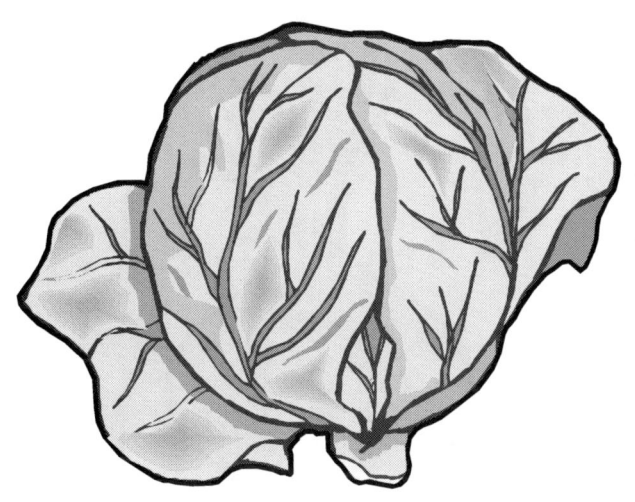

lechuga

onion

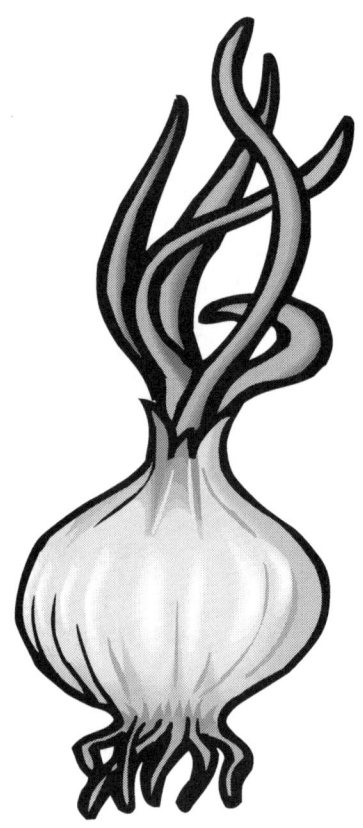

cebolla

potatoes

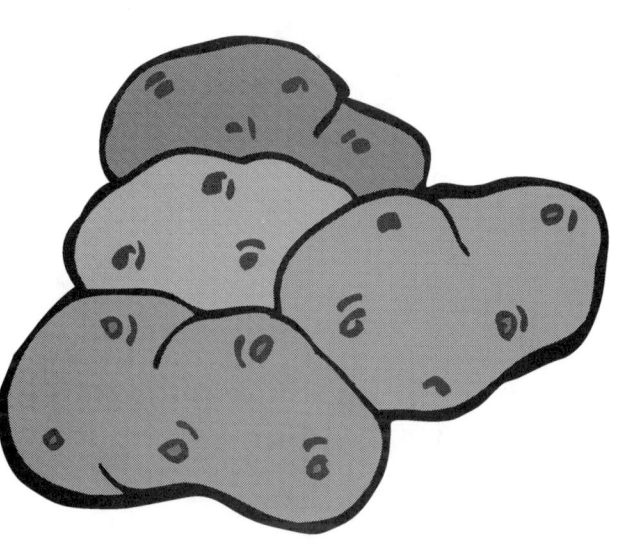

papas
also used: *patatas*

pumpkin

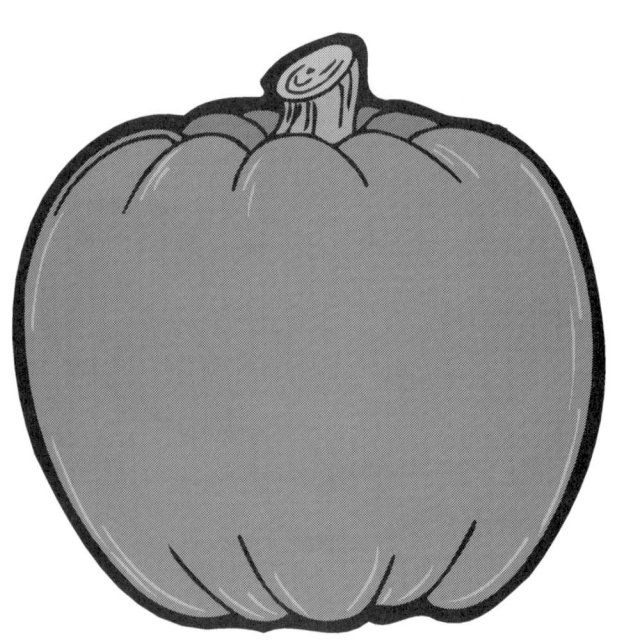

calabaza

spinach

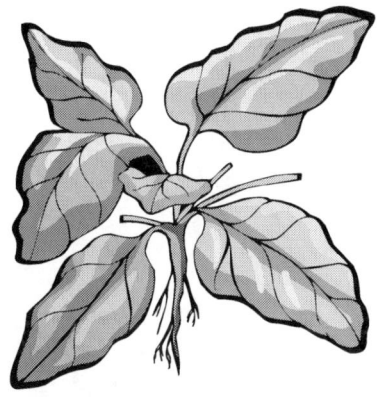

espinacas
also used: *espinaca*

tomato

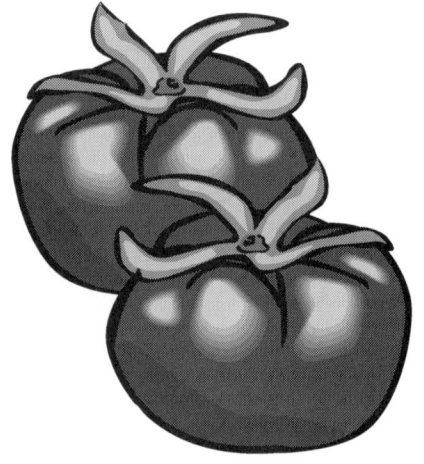

tomate
also used: *jitomate*

zucchini

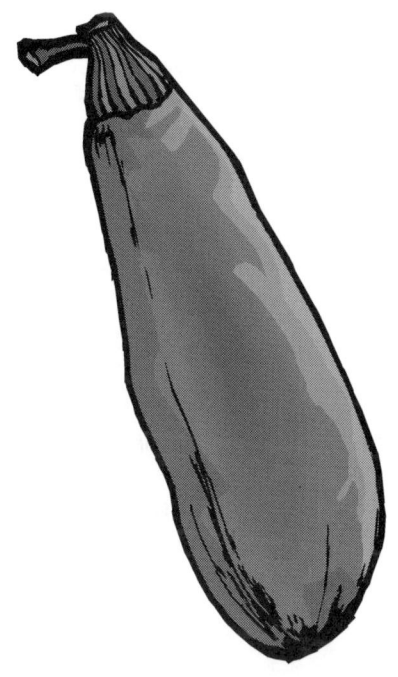

calabacita
also used: *calabacín; zapallito*

Chapter 18

Fruit

apple*	*manzana*
apricot	*albaricoque* also used: *damasco; chabacano*
banana*	*plátano* also used: *banana; banano; guineo*
blueberries*	*arándanos (azules)*
cantaloupe*	*cantalupo* also used: *melón*
cherries*	*cerezas*
cranberries	*arándanos rojos (y agrios)*
fig	*higo*
grapefruit*	*toronja** also used: *pomelo*
grapes*	*uvas*
kiwi*	*kiwi*
lemon	*limón* (Note: the Spanish words for "lemon" and "lime" vary from country to country; sometimes *lima* refers to "lemon" and *limón* refers to "lime.")
lime	*lima* also used: *limón*
mango	*mango*

Chapter includes an image of this food.

nectarine	*nectarina* also used: *pelón; durazno pelado*
orange*	*naranja* also used: *china*
papaya	*papaya*
peach*	*durazno* also used: *melocotón*
pear*	*pera*
pineapple*	*piña* also used: *ananá*
plum*	*ciruela*
raisins	*pasas* also used: *pasas de uva*
strawberry*	*fresa* also used: *frutilla*
tangerine	*mandarina*
watermelon*	*sandía* also used: *patilla*

Chapter includes an image of this food.

apple

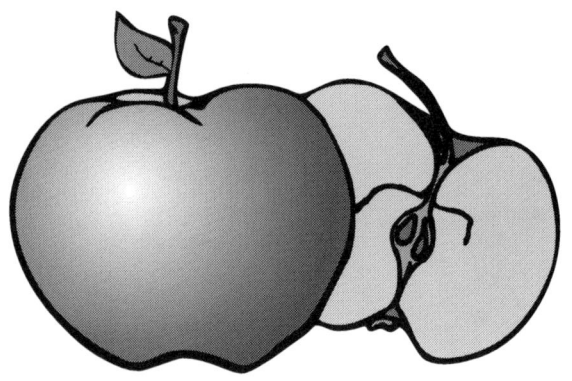

manzana

banana

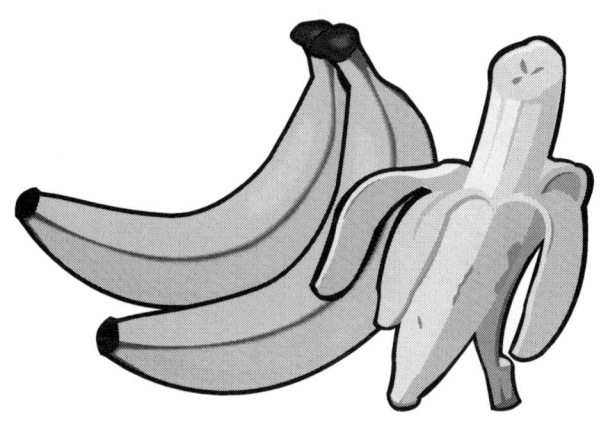

plátano
also used: *banana; banano; guineo*

blueberries

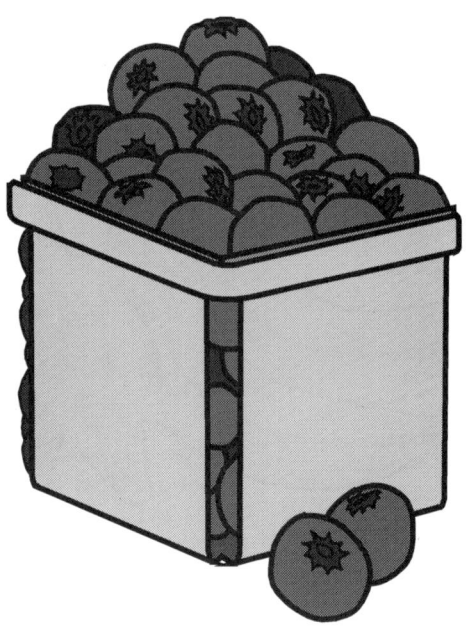

arándanos (azules)

cantaloupe

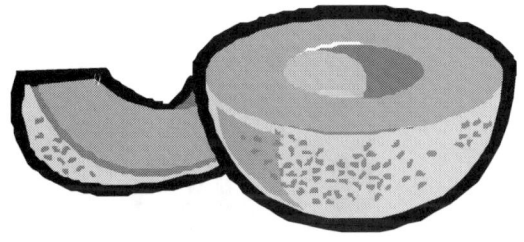

cantalupo
also used: *melón*

cherries

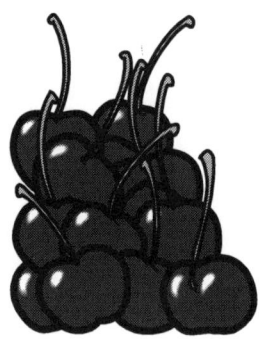

cerezas

grapefruit

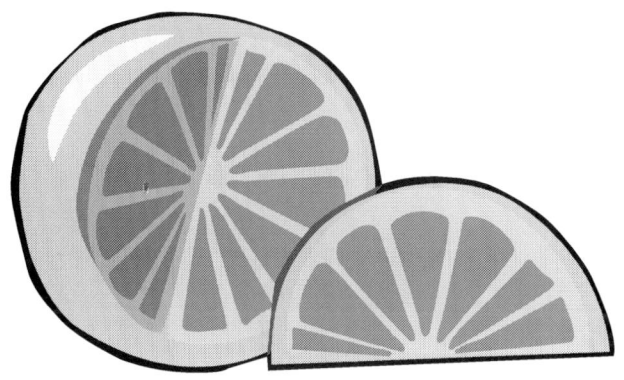

toronja
also used: *pomelo*

grapes

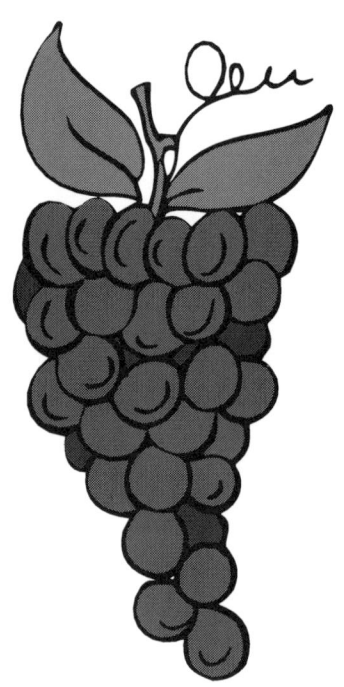

uvas

kiwi

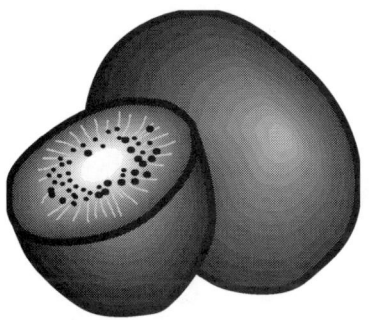

kiwi

orange

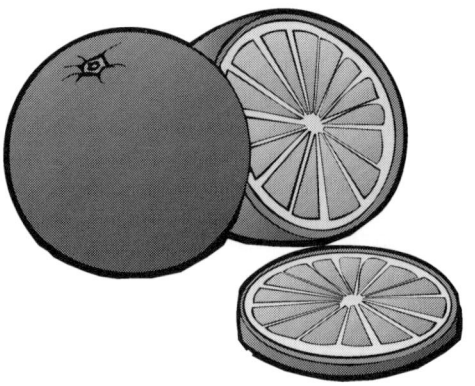

naranja
also used: *china*

peach

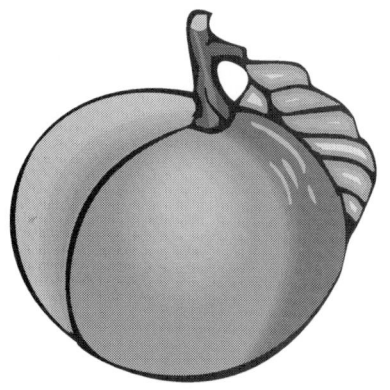

durazno
also used: *melocotón*

pear

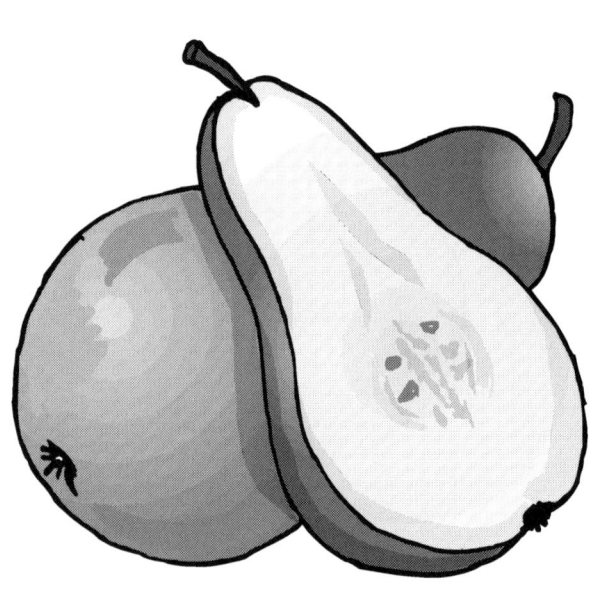

pera

pineapple

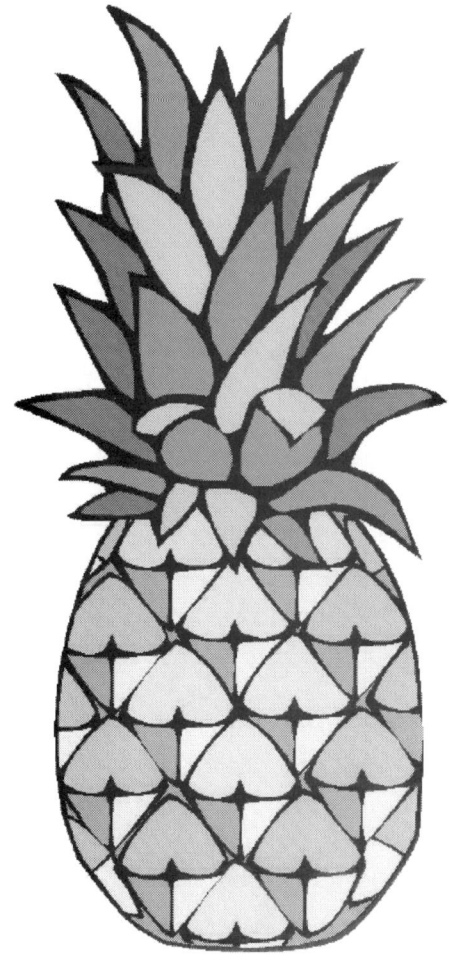

piña
also used: *ananá*

plum

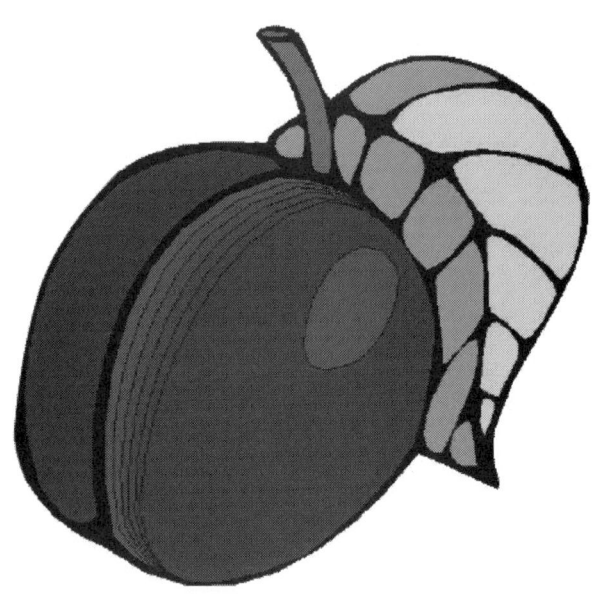

ciruela

strawberry

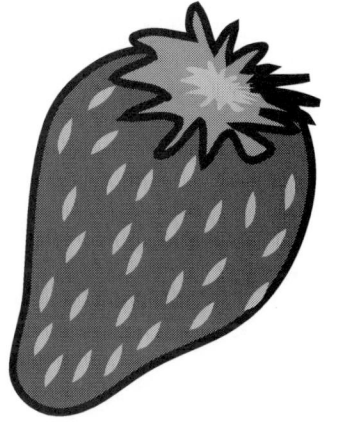

fresa
also used: *frutilla*

watermelon

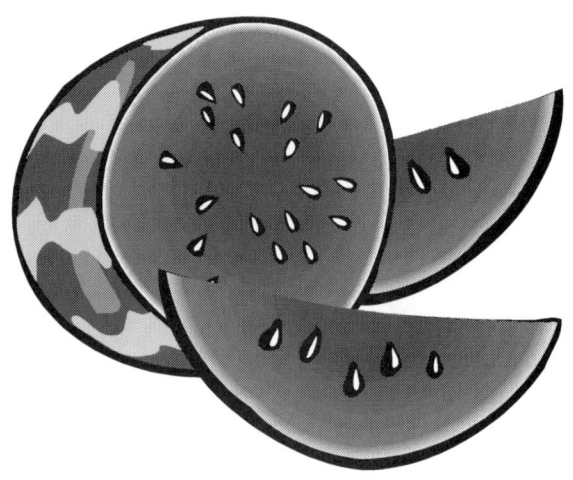

sandía
also used: *patilla*

Chapter 19

Beverages

Common Beverages

beer*	*cerveza*
coffee	*café* (for image, see Chapter 13)
coffee with milk	*café con leche*
drink/beverage	*bebida*
iced tea*	*té helado* also used: *té frío*
juice	*jugo* also used: *zumo*
apple juice	*jugo de manzana*
cranberry juice	*jugo de arándano*
fruit juice	*jugo de frutas*
grape juice	*jugo de uva*
orange juice	*jugo de naranja* also used: *jugo de china*
tomato juice	*jugo de tomate* also used: *jugo de jitomate*
vegetable juice	*jugo de verduras* also used: *jugo de vegetales*
lemonade*	*limonada*
milkshake*	*batido* also used: *licuado*
rice water	*horchata* also used: *agua de horchata*

*Chapter includes an image of this food.

smoothie	*licuado* (Note: A *licuado* is a pureed fruit drink with water, ice, and sugar, sometimes with milk and a raw egg. To describe the type of smoothie, one would say "*licuado de . . .* "—for example, *licuado de fresa* [strawberry smoothie] or *licuado de piña* [pineapple smoothie].)
soft drink	*refresco* (for image, see Chapter 14) also used: *gaseosa, soda*
diet soft drink	*refresco dieta* also used: *gaseosa dieta; refresco lite; gaseosa lite*
tea	*té*
water	*agua*
wine	*vino*
red wine	*vino tinto* also used: *vino rojo*
white wine	*vino blanco*

Varieties of Milk

(Note: For image of milk, see Chapter 13.)

buttermilk	*suero*
chocolate milk	*leche de chocolate*
cream	*crema* also used: *nata*
evaporated milk	*leche evaporada*
low-fat milk	*leche de un porciento*
nonfat milk	*leche sin grasa* also used: *leche desgrasada*

powdered milk	*leche en polvo*
reduced-fat milk	*leche de dos porciento*
sweetened condensed milk	*leche condensada*
whole milk	*leche entera* also used: *leche sin descremar*

beer

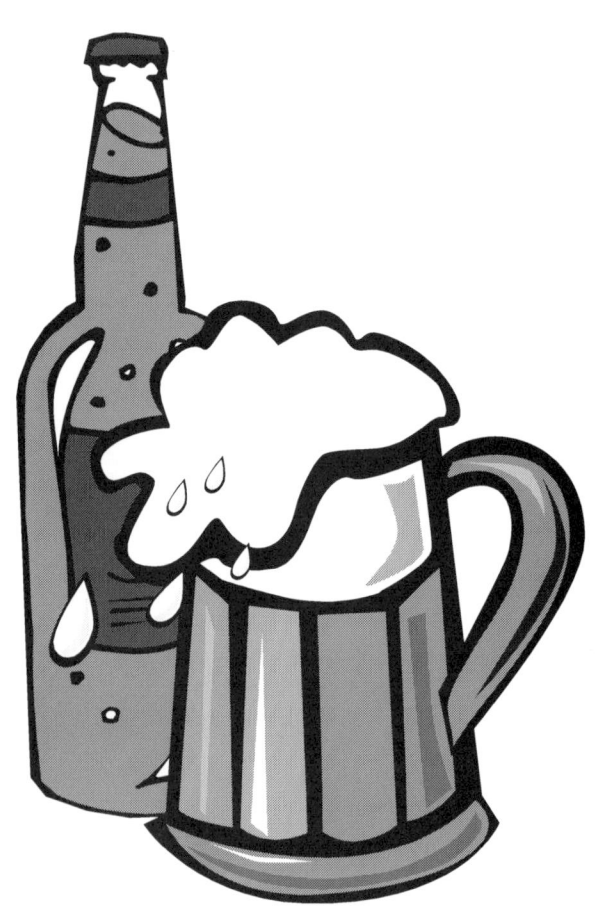

cerveza

iced tea

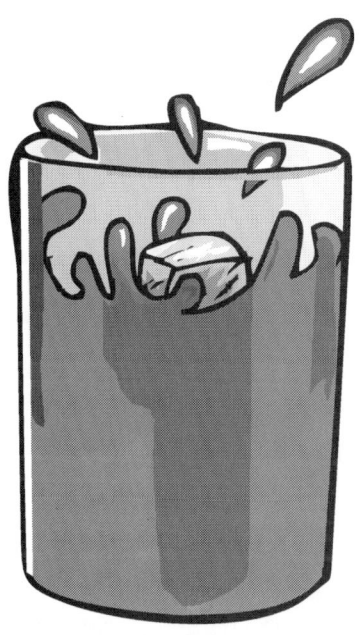

té helado
also used: *té frío*

lemonade

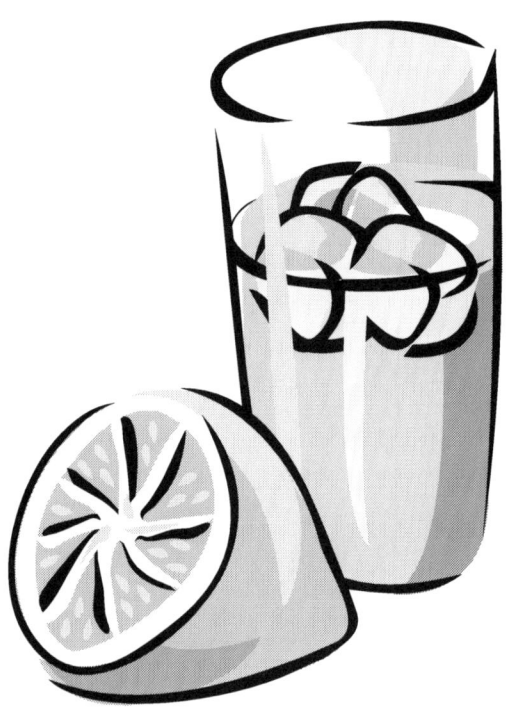

limonada

milkshake

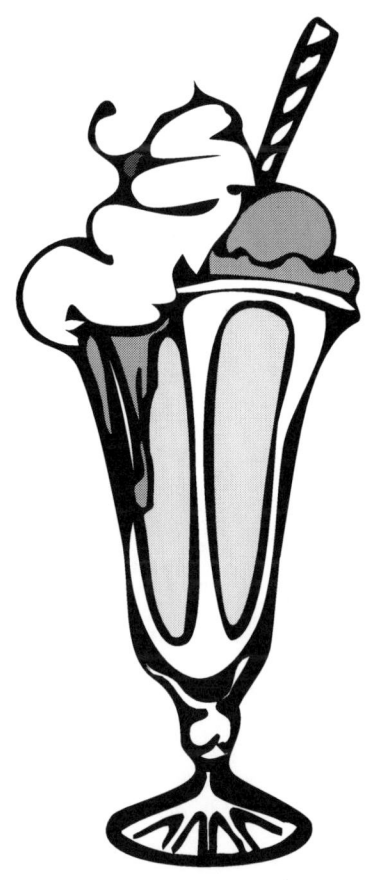

batido
also used: *licuado*

Chapter 20

Additional Foods

Cheese

American cheese	*queso americano*
blue cheese	*queso azul*
cheddar cheese	*queso cheddar*
cheese	*queso* (for image, see Chapter 13)
cottage cheese	*requesón*
fresh cheese	*queso fresco*
Monterey Jack cheese	*queso Monterey Jack*
mozzarella cheese	*queso mozzarella*
Swiss cheese	*queso suizo*
white cheese	*queso blanco*

Spices and Herbs

cilantro	*cilandro* also used: *cilantro*
cinnamon	*canela*
cumin	*comino*
garlic	*ajo*
garlic clove	*diente de ajo*
garlic salt	*sal de ajo*
nutmeg	*nuez moscada*
oregano	*orégano*
parsley	*perejil*
pepper (black)	*pimienta*

salt	*sal*
salt-free	*sin sal*
spices and herbs	*especias y hierbas*

Nuts

almonds	*almendras*
cashews	*anacardos* also used: *castaña de cajú*
hazelnuts	*avellanas*
nuts	*frutos secos* also used: *nueces*
peanuts	*cacahuates* also used: *maníes*
pecans	*pecanas* also used: *nueces*
pine nuts	*piñones*
pumpkin seeds	*pepitas*
walnuts	*nueces de Castilla* also used: *nueces; nueces de nogal*

Grains, Rice, and Flour

barley	*cebada*
bran	*salvado*
corn flour	*masa*
flour	*harina*
wheat flour	*harina de trigo* also used: *harina integral*
oats/oatmeal	*avena*
rice	*arroz*
brown rice	*arroz integral* also used: *arroz moreno*

white rice	*arroz blanco*
wild rice	*arroz silvestre*
	also used: *arroz salvaje*
whole grain	*integral*
whole wheat	*de trigo*

Oil

oil	*aceite*
olive oil	*aceite de oliva*

Chapter 21

Counseling Terms and Phrases

Introductory Conversation

What Do You Like to Eat?

In addition to knowing when (*¿cuándo?*) your clients eat, you need to know what they eat, and more importantly, what they like to eat and do not like to eat.

Question	**Possible Responses**
What do you like to eat?	I like to eat ___.
¿Qué le gusta comer (a usted)?	*Me gusta comer ___.*
What don't you like to eat?	I don't like to eat ___.
¿Qué no le gusta comer (a usted)?	*No me gusta comer ___.*
Do you like ___?	Yes, I like ___.
¿Le gusta ___?	*Sí, me gusta ___.*
	or
	No, I don't like ___.
	No, no me gusta ___.
What can't you eat?	I cannot eat dairy products.
¿Qué le hace daño?	*Me hacen daño los lácteos.*

These questions can be asked using the temporal phrases and words for meals that were listed in previous chapters. For an example, read the following dialogue between a nutrition professional (*nutricionista*) and a client (*cliente*):

Nutricionista:	*Señora Mendoza, ¿Qué le gusta comer para el desayuno?*
Cliente:	*Para el desayuno me gusta comer las frutas.*
Nutricionista:	*¿Qué frutas le gusta comer?*
Cliente:	*Me gusta mucho el mango.*
Nutricionista:	*¿Y qué no le gusta comer a usted para el desayuno?*
Cliente:	*No me gusta comer los huevos para el desayuno.*
Nutricionista:	*No me gusta comer los huevos tampoco.*

What Should I Eat? What Should I Drink?

When counseling your clients on what they should and should not eat or drink, the following questions and answers will be used frequently:

Question	Response
What should I eat?	You should eat ___.
¿Qué debo comer?	*Usted debiera comer ___.*
What should I drink?	You should drink ___.
¿Qué debo beber?	*Usted debiera beber ___.*
or	
¿Qué debo tomar?	*Usted debiera tomar ___.*
What shouldn't I eat?	You shouldn't eat ___.
¿Qué no debo comer?	*Usted no debiera comer ___.*
What shouldn't I drink?	You shouldn't drink ___.
¿Qué no debo beber?	*Usted no debiera beber ___.*
or	
¿Qué no debo tomar?	*Usted no debiera tomar ___.*

What can I eat?	You can eat ___.
¿Qué puedo comer?	*Usted puede comer ___,*

What can I drink?	You can drink ___.
¿Qué puedo beber?	*Usted puede beber ___,*

or

¿Qué puedo tomar?   *Usted puede tomar ___,*

What can't I eat?	You can't eat ___.
¿Qué no puedo comer?	*Usted no puede comer ___,*

What can't I drink?	You can't drink ___.
¿Qué no puedo beber?	*Usted no puede beber___,*

or

¿Qué no puedo tomar?   *Usted no puede tomar ___,*

What do I need to eat?	You need to eat ___.
¿Qué necesito comer?	*Usted necesita comer ___,*

What do I need to drink?	You need to drink ___.
¿Qué necesito beber?	*Usted necesita beber ___,*

or

¿Qué necesito tomar?   *Usted necesita tomar ___,*

Nutrition Guidelines

It's good to (you should) drink 8 cups of water a day.
Usted debiera beber ocho tazas de agua cada día.

or

Usted debiera tomar ocho tazas de agua cada día.

Vegetables are high in fiber and low in fat.
Las verduras son altas en fibra y bajas en grasa.

or

Las vegetales son altas en fibra y bajas en grasa.

It's good to (you should) eat ___ portions of [insert type of food].
Usted debiera comer ___ raciones de [insert type of food].

It's good to (you should) eat five fruits and vegetables a day.
Usted debiera comer cinco frutas y verduras cada día.

It would be good for you to eat every 3 hours.
Usted debiera comer cada tres horas.

Frequently Used Words and Phrases in Counseling

The following are lists of additional words and phrases you will use frequently when counseling clients. (Practice tip: Use these words and the questions and answers from the previous pages to role-play a counseling situation.)

Phrases and Terms for Use with Numbers

about or around (with time or numbers)	*más o menos*
approximately	*aproximadamente*
every ___ days	*cada ___ días*
every ___ hours	*cada ___ horas*
gram(s)	*gramo(s)*
how many?	*¿cuántos?; ¿cuántas?*
percent	*porciento*
30 percent	*el treinta por ciento*
percentage	*porcentaje*

Macronutrients and Micronutrients

calorie(s)	*caloría(s)*
carbohydrate(s)	*carbohidrato(s)*
sugar	*azúcar*
	also used: azúcares
energy	*energía*
fat	*grasa*
cholesterol	*colesterol*
saturated fat	*grasa saturada*
unsaturated fat	*grasa no saturada*
	also used: *grasa insaturada*
fiber	*fibra*
iron	*hierro*
minerals	*minerales*
phosphorus	*fósforo*
potassium	*potasio*
protein	*proteína*
sodium	*sodio*
vitamin(s)	*vitamina(s)*

Dieting and Weight

diet	*dieta*
	also used: *regimen*
to go on a diet	*ponerse a dieta*
	(or *ponerse a régimen*)
in order to gain weight	*para subir de peso; para engordarse*
in order to lose weight	*para perder peso; para bajar de peso; para adelgazar*

Other Phrases and Terms

Does it have . . . ?	*¿Tiene . . . ?*
It has . . .	*Tiene . . .*
excessive intake	*consumo excesivo*
healthy	*sano* also used: *saludable*
good for the health	*bueno/a[1] para la salud*
bad for the health	*malo/a[1] para la salud*
high in . . .	*alto/a[1] en . . .* also used: *rico/a[1] en . . .*
label	*etiqueta*
low in . . .	*bajo/a[1] en . . .*
(in) moderation	*(con) moderación*
nutritious	*nutritivo/a[1]*
servings/portions	*raciones* also used: *porciones*
too much	*demasiado/a[1]; excesivo/a[1]*

[1]*These adjectives can end in the letter "o" or the letter "a," depending on the gender of the noun that the adjective modifies. See Chapter 8 for more on this topic.*

Chapter 22

Personal Information Terms and Phrases

Personal Information about the Client

Here are some questions you may need to ask a client, and some possible answers.

Age

How old are you?
¿Cuántos años tiene usted?

I'm ___ years old.
Tengo ___ años.

Weight and Exercise

What do you usually weigh?
¿Cuánto pesa usted normalmente?

I weigh ___ pounds.
Peso ___ libras.

How much weight have you gained?
¿Cuánto peso ha aumentado?

What was your pre-pregnancy weight?
¿Cuánto pesaba usted antes de salir embarazada?

Do you exercise?
¿Hace usted ejercicio?

For how long?
¿Por cuánto tiempo?

How many days per week?
¿Cuántos días a la semana?

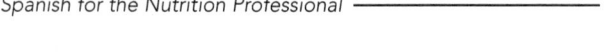
Cultural Tidbit

Most Spanish-speaking countries use the metric system and measure body weight in kilograms (*kilos*). If the answer to the question "How much do you weigh?" seems very low, the client is probably stating his or her weight in kilograms. The conversion is as follows:

Weight in pounds/2.2 = Weight in kilograms

Family History

Does diabetes run in your family?
¿Tiene familiares con diabetes?

Does heart disease run in your family?
¿Tiene familiares con enfermedad de corazón?

Medication Use

Do you take any medications?   Yes, I take ___.
¿Toma usted medicamentos?   *Sí, tomo ___.*

or

¿Toma usted medicinas?

Alcohol Intake

How many alcoholic drinks do you have per day?
¿Cuántas bebidas alcohólicas toma al día?

How many alcoholic drinks do you have per week?
¿Cuántas bebidas alcohólicas toma a la semana?

Dairy Intake

Do you drink milk?
¿Bebe usted leche? or *¿Toma usted leche?*

What kind?
¿Qué clase? or *¿Qué tipo?* or *¿De cuál?*

Are you lactose intolerant?
¿Tiene usted intolerancia a la lactosa?

Diseases and Conditions

You can use the following vocabulary to discuss diseases or conditions your client may have.

Diseases and Disorders

Do you have ___? *¿Tiene usted___ ?*	I have ___. *Tengo ___,*
anemia	*anemia*
anorexia (nervosa)	*anorexia (nerviosa)*
bulimia (nervosa)	*bulimia (nerviosa)*
constipation	*estreñimiento*
diabetes	*diabetes*
diarrhea	*diarrea*
(a) disease	*(una) enfermedad*
(a) disorder	*(un) trastorno*
gestational diabetes	*diabetes gestacional* also used: *diabetes del embarazo*
gluten allergy	*alergia al gluten*
headaches	*dolores de cabeza*
high blood pressure	*presión (arterial) alta* also used: *alta presión*
high cholesterol	*colesterol alto*
hunger	*hambre*
lactose intolerance	*intolerancia a la lactosa*
liver disease	*enfermedad del hígado*
low blood pressure	*presión (arterial) baja* also used: *baja presión*
malnutrition	*desnutrición*

nausea	*náuseas*
obesity	*obesidad*
overweight	*sobrepeso*
renal disease	*enfermedad renal* also used: *enfermedad de los riñones*
thirst	*sed*

Food Allergies

Do you have any food allergies?
¿Le hace daño algún alimento?

or

¿Tiene usted alérgias a algún alimento?

Eating Disorders

Are you ___?	I am ___.
¿Es usted ___?	*Soy ___.*
anorexic	*anoréxico/a[1]*
bulimic	*bulímico/a[1]*

Pregnancy

Are you pregnant?	*¿Está usted embarazada?*
I'm pregnant.	*Estoy embarazada.*

---

[1] *These adjectives can end in the letter "o" or the letter "a," depending on the gender of the person with the condition. See Chapter 8 for more on this topic.*

Personal Information Terms and Phrases

Questions the Client May Ask

How many calories does ___ have?
¿Cuántas calorías tiene ___?

[Insert food name] has [insert number] calories.
[Insert food name] *tiene* [insert number] *calorías.*

Should I lose weight?
¿Debo perder peso?

Chapter 23

Cooking and Recipe Terms

Methods of Preparation

The following terms refer to cooking and recipes and can be useful in discussing food preparation with your client.

baked	*al horno* also used: *horneado/a*[1]
boiled	*hervido/a*[1]
broiled	*a la parilla* also used: *asado/a*[1]
canned	*en lata* also used: *enlatado/a*[1]
chopped	*picado/a*[1]
cooked	*cocido/a*[1]
cut up	*cortado/a*[1]
fat-free	*sin grasa*
fresh	*fresco/a*[1]
fried	*frito/a*[1]
not breaded, not fried	*ni empanizado/a*[1], *ni frito/a*[1]
frozen	*congelado/a*[1]
grilled	*asado/a*[1]
low-fat	*bajo/a*[1] *en grasa*
microwaved	*cocido/a*[1] *en microondas*
prepared	*preparado/a*[1]

[1] *These adjectives can end in the letter "o" or the letter "a," depending on the gender of the noun that the adjective modifies. See Chapter 8 for more on this topic.*

raw	*crudo/a[1]*
salt-free	*sin sal*
with less salt	*con menos sal*
sautéed	*sofrito/a[1]*
	also used: *salteado/a[1]*
served	*servido/a[1]*
skim	*descremado/a[1]*
sliced	*rebanado/a[1]*
	also used: *tajado/a[1]*
spread	*untado/a[1]*
steamed	*cocido/a[1] al vapor*
stewed	*guisado/a[1]*
stir-fried	*sofrito/a[1]*
sugar-free	*sin azúcar*
well-done	*bien hecho/a[1]*
	also used: *bien cocido/a[1]*
with	*con*
without	*sin*

Portion and Measurement Terms

clove (of garlic)	*diente (de ajo)*
cube(s)	*cubo(s)*
cup(s)	*taza(s)*
half	*media*
	also used: *mitad*
less	*menos*
more	*más*
ounce(s)	*onza(s)*
piece(s)	*trozo(s)*
	also used: *pedazo(s)*
small piece(s)	*trocito(s)*
	also used: *pedacito(s)*

[1]*These adjectives can end in the letter "o" or the letter "a," depending on the gender of the noun that the adjective modifies. See Chapter 8 for more on this topic.*

strip(s)	*tira(s)*
	also used: *rodaja(s)*
tablespoon	*cucharada*
teaspoon	*cucharadita*

Section III

Nutrition Care
Education and Resources

Chapter 24

Nutrition Education and the Non-English-Speaking Client

Health Literacy and Nutrition Education

The 1992 National Adult Literacy Survey conducted by the U.S. government showed that almost half of Americans read at basic levels (eighth-grade level or below) and another 22 million lack the ability to read (1). The basic readers include 76 percent of older adults, 66 percent of people living in poverty, 76 percent of people with chronic health conditions, and two-thirds of ethnic minorities (1).

Although the average reading level in the United States is at about a sixth-grade level, most health information (including nutrition education material) is written at above the tenth-grade level. In addition, educators, including nutrition professionals, tend to overestimate their clients' abilities and underestimate the complexity of the materials they use (2).

Health literacy is defined by the American Medical Association as "the ability to read, understand, and act on health care information," and literacy is the single best predictor of health status (3). Communicating nutrition and health information can be even more challenging when the nutrition professional and the client do not speak the same language. In addition, clients who are able to communicate socially in English often do not have the language skills to understand nutrition and health issues (4).

If you use materials that your client cannot easily read, your client may not understand your message and may feel distrust or anger. Your client may not be able to take the actions you recommend and, thus, may not see the value of nutrition counseling (2). In addition, client education material that is not reading-level appropriate may place you out of compliance with federal mandates (1998) to use "plain language" as well as the Joint Commission on Accreditation of Healthcare Organizations (JCAHO) standards for patient and family education, which hold institutions accountable for providing culturally appropriate information that is understandable to clients who receive it (5,6).

Stress, illness, pain, and some medications reduce the ability to read, learn, and remember; and many well-educated people have difficulty with health and nutrition terms and concepts (7). Coping skills that allow a poor reader to function at work may not work when there is an urgent health problem. Low health literacy is estimated to cost health care systems $50 billion to $73 billion annually (8).

Designing, Selecting, or Adapting Easy-to-Read Materials

You may have difficulty finding culturally appropriate materials for your Latino clients (9). Some materials may contain useful information but may not be written in an easy-to-read format (10). You may find that you need to design or adapt materials and resources.

Most education materials contain too much information. Giving more information to clients with the hope that at least some of it will be retained has the opposite effect—the more information given to clients, the less they remember. Concentrating on just the key (essential) messages will enhance retention and learning (7).

Designing easy-to-read material is more involved than simply writing to a lower reading level. A brief overview of the attributes of easy-to-read material follows. See the resource list for more information.

Creating Content

The following are suggestions for creating content for easy-to-read educational materials (2,3,7):

- Limit content to three to five key messages. Adults have difficulty remembering more than five new "facts." Focus on "need to know" information rather than "nice to know" information because information overload does not enhance learning.
- Use simple words. See the list in the table below (11).
- Make sure the content of the material is age appropriate and reflects your client's culture.

Using Easy-to-Read Words

Instead of. . .	Try . . .	Instead of. . .	Try . . .
Absence of	No, none	Function	Work, do
Accomplish	Do	Guidelines	Steps to follow, directions
Accurate	Right		
Additional	More	Identify	Show, name, find
Acquire	Get	Implement	Do, follow
Alternative	Choice	Information	Facts
Approximately	About	Large numbers of	Many, most
Attempt	Try	Maintain	Keep, look after, save
Benefit	Help	Modify	Change
Consider	Think about	Monitor	Check on, watch
Consult	Ask, check with, talk to	Notify	Call, tell, let us know
Contains	Has	Objective	Aim, goal, what we hope to do
Correct	Right		
Currently	Now	Purchase	Buy
Deficiency	Lack	Recommend	Suggest, guide
Discontinue	Stop, end, quit	Requirement	Need
Disturbance	Problem, change	Restriction	Limit
Effect	Make	Select	Choose
Encourage	Ask to, help	Supply	Give
Ensure	Make sure	Urgent	Cannot wait long
Exceed	Go beyond, pass	Utilize	Use
Explain	Tell, show		
Factor	Cause	*Source: Adapted from Federal Aviation*
Feasible	Can be done, will work	*Administration. Writing user-friendly*
Finalize	Finish up, end	*documents. Available at:*
For further instructions	Find out what to do next	*http://www.faa.gov/language/docs/ guidance2.htm. Accessed August 26, 2004.*

Writing Text

Tips for writing successful educational materials include the following (2,7,10):

- Use one of the many available resources to ensure that reading level is sixth grade or below, if appropriate. (See the resource list.)
- Use one- or two-syllable words whenever possible ("show" instead of "demonstrate").
- Use shorter sentences. For example, a sentence should be no more than 10 to 15 words.
- Use strong, direct language; do not use passive voice. For example, use "Your dietitian will weigh you" instead of "You will be weighed by the dietitian." (Note that a culturally sensitive translation may change some language patterns.)
- Be careful not to turn verbs into nouns. For example, use "predicted" instead of "made the prediction."
- Do not use unnecessary words or phrases. For example, use "This supplement may upset your stomach" instead of "This supplement may cause you to experience nausea."
- Keep the information personal. For example, write "Take your vitamins when you eat a meal."
- Use specific examples instead of abstract ideas. For example, write "Read the label. Make sure your cereal has at least six grams of fiber in a half-cup serving" instead of "Choose a high-fiber cereal."
- Paragraphs should be short with only a single key message in each.

Incorporating Fonts

Some typefaces are easier to read than others. Here is some guidance for working with fonts (2,7,10):

- Use one of the more readable fonts, such as Garamond, Bembo, or Times. Do not incorporate more than two or three font styles on a page.
- Use uppercase and lowercase text. Many poor readers recognize words by sight, and uppercase words may run together and look the same.
- Use a minimum of 12-point font with serifs.

Layout and Design

Good design helps the reader. Consider the following techniques when designing educational material (2,3,7):

- Make sure the margins are wide enough and that there is enough white space. Avoid too much text or clutter.
- Separate blocks of text with headings and subheadings.
- Use bulleted lists when possible.
- Use a two-column layout.
- Justify the text on the left, but not the right. Uneven spacing between words can make reading more difficult for your client.
- Choose black or dark blue ink on white or cream-colored paper. This combination (contrast) is easiest to read.
- Incorporate illustrations only if they are useful additions to the content. Also, keep in mind that images of individuals should represent your intended audience.

Tips for Creating or Selecting Culturally Appropriate Materials

To be effective, educational materials must suit their audiences. Keep in mind the following points when creating or selecting materials for Latino clients:

- Materials should include words Latino clients know (2). Include the English version of key words so clients can begin to learn about foods in the United States.
- Your recommendations should be consistent with your client's lifestyle. For example, discuss salsa rather than another condiment (10).
- Field-test materials with Latino clients. Listen to what they say. They will be the best judges of what is useful and appropriate. If possible, solicit opinions one-on-one or in focus groups to improve your materials (2).
- When materials are translated, ensure that each is as simple and as easy as possible to follow. Your translator should understand basic nutrition terms and concepts. Also, as stated above, incorporate suggestions that will make the translated material easy to read. Another tip: ask that the material be translated back into English to ensure that the

original message is accurate (7,9).

- If your intended audience consists of more than one Latino group, be certain to incorporate alternate words wherever possible. For example, depending on their country of origin, clients may use *los guisantes, los chicharos,* or *las arvejas* for "peas."
- Audiotapes, videotapes, and DVDs can be useful for clients who are poor readers or have other difficulties (9).

References

1. Kirsch IS, Jungeblut A, Jenkins L, Kolstad A. *Executive Summary of Adult Literacy in America: A First Look at the Results of the National Adult Literacy Survey.* Washington, DC: National Center for Education Statistics, US Department of Education; 1993.

2. Root J, Stableford S. *Write It Easy-to-Read: A Guide to Creating Plain English Materials.* Biddeford, Me: University of New England; 1998.

3. Weiss B. *Health Literacy: A Manual for Clinicians.* Chicago, Ill: American Medical Association; 2003.

4. Osborne H. *Overcoming Communication Barriers in Patient Education.* Gaithersburg, Md: Aspen Publishers; 2001.

5. Plain language in government writing. *Fed Register.* 1998;63:31885-31886. Available at: http://www.mrm.mms.gov/laws_R_D/FRNotices/ PDFDocs/31885.pdf. Accessed September 3, 2004.

6. *Accreditation Manual for Hospitals and Healthcare Organizations: Provision of Care, Treatment, and Services.* Chicago, Ill: Joint Commission on Accreditation of Healthcare Organizations; 2004.

7. Doak C, Doak L, Root J. *Teaching Patients with Low Literacy Skills.* 2nd ed. Philadelphia, Pa: JB Lippincott; 1996.

8. Friedland R. *Understanding Health Literacy: New Estimates of the Costs of Inadequate Health Literacy.* Washington, DC: National Academy on an Aging Society; 1998.

9. Curry K, Jaffe, A. *Nutrition Counseling and Communication Skills.* Philadelphia, Pa: WB Saunders; 1998.

10. *Beyond the Brochure: Alternative Approaches to Effective Health Communication.* Denver, Colo: AMC Cancer Research Center; 1994. Available at: http://www.cdc.gov/cancer/nbccedp/bccpdfs/amcbeyon. pdf. Accessed September 3, 2004.

11. Federal Aviation Administration. Writing user-friendly documents. Available at: http://www.faa.gov/language/ docs/guidance2.htm. Accessed August 26, 2004.

Chapter 25

Selected Resources for the Nutrition Professional

Hispanic Culture and Health Statistics

Diversity Rx. Available at: http://www.diversityrx.org. Accessed October 25, 2004.

National Alliance for Hispanic Health Web site. Available at: http://www.hispanichealth.org. Accessed October 25, 2004.

Office of Minority Health Resources Center Web site. Available at: http://www.omhrc.gov. Accessed October 25, 2004.

Evaluating the Reading Level of Materials

Doak C, Doak L, Root J. *Teaching Patients with Low Literacy Skills.* 2nd ed. Philadelphia, Pa: JB Lippincott; 1996.

The SMOG Readability Formula. (Explains Suitability Assessment of Materials Scoring [SMOG].) Available at: http://www.med.utah.edu/pated/authors/readability.html. Accessed September 3, 2004.

Food and Nutrition

Ethnic Foods Nutrient Composition Guide. 2nd ed. Sunnyvale, Calif: Four Winds Food Specialists; 2001.

Kittler P, Sucher K. *Food and Culture.* 4th ed. Belmont, Calif: Wadsworth Publishing; 2003.

National Dairy Council. Lactose Intolerance and Minorities: The Real Story. Available at: http://nationaldairycouncil.org/nutrition/lactose/lactoseIntolerance.pdf. Accessed October 12, 2004.

Raichlen S. *Healthy Latin Cooking.* New York: Rodale Press; 1998.

Rodriguez JC. *Contemporary Nutrition for Latinos.* Lincoln, Neb: iUniverse; 2004.

University of Texas Health Science Center. Hispanic Americans and Health Bibliographies. Available at: http://www.library.uthscsa.edu/basics/hisbib.cfm. Accessed October 12, 2004.

Health Literacy

Harvard School of Public Health Health Literacy Studies Web site. Available at: http://www.hsph.harvard.edu/healthliteracy. Accessed October 25, 2004.

Oregon State University Extension Family and Community Development. Readable materials. Available at: http://extension.oregonstate.edu/fcd/nutrition/commprograms/readablematerial/index.php. Accessed October 27, 2004.

Plain Language Web site. Available at: http://www.plainlanguage.gov. Accessed October 25, 2004.

Wisconsin Nutrition Education Program. Teaching Resources for Spanish Language. http://www.uwex.edu/ces/wnep/tch_res/res_list.cfm?language_id=2. Accessed October 27, 2004.

Health Information Resources for Latino Clients

Food Guide Pyramid with a Mexican Flavor, Lesson Plan: Pirámide del día con el sabor popular mexicano. Oakland, Calif: University of California Agriculture and Natural Resources Communication Services; 1999. To purchase: call 800/998.8849 (product code 33904).

Hispanic Health Council. Bilingual Puerto Rican food guide pyramid [poster]. Available at: http://hispanichealth.com/material.html. Accessed October 12, 2004.

Hispanic Health Council. Bilingual food label. Available at: http://hispanic health.com/material.html. Accessed October 12, 2004.

National Heart, Lung, and Blood Institute. Latino cardiovascular health resources. Available at: http://www.nhlbi.nih.gov/health/prof/heart/latino/lat_8pub.htm. Accessed October 27, 2004.

Oregon State University Extension Family and Community Development. Readable materials. Available at: http://extension.oregonstate.edu/fcd/nutrition/commprograms/readablematerial/index.php. Accessed October 27, 2004.

US Department of Agriculture Food and Nutrition Information Center. Food guide pyramid: ethnic/cultural. Available at: http://www.nal.usda.gov/fnic/etext/000023.html. Accessed October 12, 2004.

US Department of Agriculture Food and Nutrition Information Center. Index of ethnic and cultural resources. Available at: http://www.nal.usda.gov/fnic/etext/000010.html. Accessed October 12, 2004.

US Food and Drug Administration. Easy-to-read publications. Available at: http://www.fda.gov/opacom/lowlit/7lowlit.html. Accessed October 27, 2004.

Wisconsin Nutrition Education Program. Teaching Resources for Spanish Language. http://www.uwex.edu/ces/wnep/tch_res/res_list.cfm?language_id=2.

Glossary

A

about or around (with time or numbers)	*más o menos*
after	*después (de)*
afternoon	*tarde*
alcoholic beverages	*bebidas alcohólicas*
allergy	*alergia*
almonds	*almendras*
always	*siempre*
(I) am	*(yo) soy; (yo) estoy*
and	*y*
anemia	*anemia*
anorexia (nervosa)	*anorexia (nerviosa)*
anorexic	*anoréxico/a*
appetizer	*bocadillo*
apple	*manzana*
apple juice	*jugo de manzana*
approximately	*aproximadamente*
apricot	*albaricoque; damasco; chabacano*
artificial sweetner	*endulzante (artificial)*
at	*a*
avacado	*aguacate*

B

bacon	*tocino; tocineta; panceta*
bad	*mal; malo/a*
bad for the health	*malo/a para la salud*
baked	*al horno; horneado/a*
banana	*plátano; banana; banano; guineo*
barley	*cebada*
beans, dried	*frijoles; habichuelas; porotos*
beans, green	*judías verdes*
because	*porque*
beef	*carne de res; carne roja*
beer	*cerveza*
before	*antes (de)*
beverage	*bebida*
blood pressure	*presión (arterial)*
blueberries	*arándanos (azules)*
boiled	*hervido/a*
bran	*salvado*
bread	*pan*
bread, wheat	*pan de trigo*
bread, white	*pan blanco*
bread, whole-grain	*pan integral*
bread roll	*bolillo; panecillo*
breaded	*empanizado/a*
bread pudding	*capirotada*
breakfast	*desayuno*
broccoli	*brócoli; brécol*
broiled	*asado/a; a la parilla*
brussels sprouts	*col de Bruselas; Bruselas; repollitos de Bruselas; colecitas de Bruselas*

bulimia (nervosa)	*bulimia (nerviosa)*
bulimic	*bulímico/a*
but	*pero; sino*
butter	*mantequilla; manteca*
buttermilk	*suero*

C

cabbage	*col; repollo*
cactus	*nopal; nopalitos*
cake	*pastel; torta; biscocho*
calorie(s)	*caloría(s)*
can (noun)	*lata*
(I) can	*(yo) puedo*
(you) can	*(usted) puede*
candy; sweets	*dulces; caramelos; golosinas*
canned	*en lata; enlatado/a*
(I) cannot	*(yo) no puedo*
(you) cannot	*(usted) no puede*
cantaloupe	*cantalupo, melón*
carbohydrate(s)	*carbohidrato(s)*
carrots	*zanahorias*
cashews	*anacardos; castaña de cajú*
cauliflower	*coliflor*
cereal	*cereal; maizoro*
cheese	*queso*
cheese, American	*queso americano*
cheese, blue	*queso azul*
cheese, cheddar	*queso cheddar*
cheese, cottage	*requesón*
cheese, fresh	*queso fresco*
cheese, Monterey Jack	*queso Monterey Jack*

cheese, mozzarella	*queso mozzarella*
cheese, Swiss	*queso suizo*
cheese, white	*queso blanco*
cherries	*cerezas*
chicken	*pollo*
chips (snack)	*chips; totopos; papitas de bolsa; papitas fritas; tostaditas*
chocolate	*chocolate*
cholesterol	*colesterol*
chopped	*picado/a*
cilantro	*cilandro; cilantro*
cinnamon	*canela*
client	*cliente*
clove of garlic	*diente de ajo*
codfish	*bacalao*
coffee	*café*
coffee with milk	*café con leche*
cold cuts	*carne para sándwich*
cole slaw	*ensalada de col; ensalada de repollo*
condition	*condición*
constipation	*estreñimiento*
cooked	*cocido/a*
cookies	*galletas dulces*
corn	*maíz*
corn flour	*masa*
corn on the cob	*elote; mazorca de maíz; choclo de maíz*
cottage cheese	*requesón*
country	*país*
crackers	*galletas saladas*
cranberries	*arándanos rojos (y agrios)*

cranberry juice	*jugo de arándano*
cream	*crema; nata*
cube(s)	*cubo(s)*
cucumber	*pepino*
cumin	*comino*
cup(s)	*taza(s)*
cupcake	*pastelito; magdalena; cubilete; mantecada; pastelillo*
custard	*flan*
cut up	*cortado/a*

D

dairy products	*lácteos*
days	*días*
desserts	*postres*
diabetes	*diabetes*
diarrhea	*diarrea*
diet	*dieta; régimen*
(to) diet	*ponerse a dieta; ponerse a régimen*
diet soft drink	*refresco dieta; gaseosa dieta; refresco lite; gaseosa lite*
dinner	*cena*
disease	*enfermedad*
disorders	*trastornos*
donuts	*donas; rosquillas*
drink (noun)	*bebida*
(I) drink	*bebo; tomo*
(to) drink	*beber; tomar*
(you) drink	*bebe; toma*

E

(I) eat	*como*
(you) eat	*come*
eggs	*huevos; blanquillos*
egg white	*clara de huevo; clara de blanquillo*
egg yolk	*yema de huevo; yema de blanquillo*
energy	*energía*
English	*inglés*
every day	*cada día; todos los días*
excessive intake	*consumo excesivo*
exercise	*ejercicio*

F

family members	*familiares*
fat	*grasa*
fat-free	*sin grasa*
fiber	*fibra*
fig	*higo*
fine	*bien*
fish	*pescado*
flour (white)	*harina*
flour, wheat	*harina de trigo; harina integral*
food	*comida; alimento*
food allergy	*alergia alimenticia*
for	*por; para*
french fries	*papas fritas; papitas*
french toast	*torrija; torreja*
fresh	*fresco/a*

fried	*frito/a*
fried pork skins	*chicharrones*
fritters	*buñuelos; sopaipillas*
from	*de*
frozen	*congelado/a*
fruit juice	*jugo de frutas*
fruits	*frutas*

G

(to) gain weight	*(para) subir de peso; (para) engordarse*
garlic	*ajo*
garlic clove	*diente de ajo*
garlic salt	*sal de ajo*
gelatin	*gelatina*
generally	*generalmente*
gestational diabetes	*diabetes gestacional; diabetes del embarazo*
gluten allergy	*alergia al gluten*
good afternoon	*buenas tardes*
good-bye	*adiós*
good for the health	*bueno/a para la salud*
good evening	*buenas noches*
good morning	*buenos días*
good night	*buenas noches*
grams	*gramos*
grapefruit	*toronja; pomelo*
grape juice	*jugo de uva*
grapes	*uvas*
green beans	*judías verdes; ejotes; porotos verdes; habichuelas*

green leafy vegetables	*verduras de hojas verdes*
grilled	*asado/a; a la parilla*
grilled cheese sandwich	*sándwich de queso fundido*
ground beef	*carne molida; carne picada*

H

half	*media; mitad*
half past	*y media*
ham	*jamón*
hamburger	*hamburguesa*
(it) has	*tiene*
hash browns	*papas doradas*
(I) have	*(yo) tengo*
(you) have	*(usted) tiene*
hazelnuts	*avellanas*
headaches	*dolores de cabeza*
healthy	*sano; saludable*
heart disease	*enfermedad de corazón*
hello	*hola*
herbs	*hierbas*
high blood pressure	*presión (arterial) alta; alta presión*
high cholesterol	*colesterol alto*
high in	*alto/a en; rico/a en*
honey	*miel de abeja*
hot chocolate	*chocolate*
hot dog	*hot dog; pancho; salchica*
hour	*hora*
How are you?	*¿Cómo está usted?*
how many	*cuántos; cuántas*
how much	*cuánto/a*

How old are you?	*¿Cuántos años tiene usted?*
hunger	*hambre*
(I'm) hungry	*tengo hambre*
(you're) hungry	*tiene hambre*

I

I	*yo*
ice cream	*helado; nieve*
iced tea	*té helado; té frío*
if	*si*
I'm sorry	*lo siento; disculpe*
in	*en*
iron	*hierro*

J

jelly	*jalea; mermelada; dulce*
jicama	*jícama*
juice	*jugo; zumo*

K

ketchup	*catsup; salsa de tomate; salsa de jitomate*
kidney disease	*enfermedad renal*
kilogram	*kilogramo; kilo*
kiwi	*kiwi*

L

label	*etiqueta*
lactose intolerance	*intolerancia a la lactosa*
lay healer	*curandero*
legumes	*leguminosas*
lemon	*limón; lima*

lemonade	*limonada*
less	*menos*
lettuce	*lechuga*
(I) like	*me gusta*
(you) like	*le gusta*
lime	*lima; limón*
liver	*hígado*
liver disease	*enfermedad del hígado*
(to) lose weight	*(para) perder peso; (para) bajar de peso; (para) adelgazar*
low blood pressure	*presión (arterial) baja; baja presión*
low-fat	*bajo/a en grasa*
low in	*bajo/a en*
lunch	*almuerzo; comida; lonche*

M

malnutrition	*desnutrición*
mango	*mango*
many	*mucho/a*
margarine	*margarina*
mayonnaise	*mayonesa*
meal	*comida*
meat, red	*carne roja*
medications	*medicamentos; medicinas*
microwaved	*cocido/a en microondas*
milk	*leche*
milk, chocolate	*leche de chocolate*
milk, evaporated	*leche evaporada*
milk, low-fat (1%)	*leche de un porciento*

milk, nonfat (skim)	*leche sin grasa; leche desgrasada*
milk, powdered	*leche en polvo*
milk, reduced-fat (2%)	*leche de dos porciento*
milk, sweetened condensed	*leche condensada*
milk, whole	*leche entera; leche sin descremar*
milkshake	*batido; licuado*
minerals	*minerales*
minute	*minuto*
Miss	*Señorita*
(in) moderation	*(con) moderación*
more	*más*
morning	*la mañana*
Mr.	*Señor*
Mrs.	*Señora*
muffin	*panque; panecillo; mollete; muffin*
mustard	*mostaza*
My name is …	*Me llamo …*

N

name	*nombre*
nausea	*náuseas*
nectarine	*nectarina; pelón, durazno pelado*
(I) need	*necesito*
(to) need	*necesitar*
(you) need	*necesita*
neither	*tampoco*
never	*nunca*
night	*noche*
no	*no*
noodles	*fideos*
nor	*ni*

normally	*normalmente*
not breaded or fried	*ni empanizado/a ni frito/a*
number	*número* (for specific numbers, see Chapter 10)
nutmeg	*nuez moscada*
nutrition professional	*nutricionista*
nutritious	*nutritivo/a*
nuts	*frutos secos; nueces*

O

oats/oatmeal	*avena*
obesity	*obesidad*
of	*de*
oil	*aceite*
olive oil	*aceite de oliva*
on	*en*
onion	*cebolla*
or	*o*
orange	*naranja; china*
orange juice	*jugo de naranja; jugo de china*
oregano	*orégano*
ounce(s)	*onza(s)*
overweight	*sobrepeso*

P

pancakes	*panqueques; panques; crepas; panquecas; hotcakes*
papaya	*papaya*
parsley	*perejil*
pasta	*pasta*
pastry	*pan dulce*
peach	*durazno; melocotón*

peanut butter	*crema de cacahuate; crema de maní; mantequilla de cacahuate; mantequilla de maní*
peanuts	*cacahuates; manies*
pear	*pera*
peas, green	*guisantes; chícharos; petit pois; arvejas*
peas, pigeon	*gandules*
pecans	*pecanas; nueces*
pepper, black	*pimienta*
pepper, green bell	*pimiento verde; chile verde; aji verde; chile ancho*
percent	*porciento*
percentage	*porcentaje*
phosphorus	*fósforo*
pie	*pai; pastel; empanada; tarta; torta*
pieces	*trozos; pedazos*
pineapple	*piña; ananá*
pine nuts	*piñones*
pizza	*pizza*
plantain	*plátano; plátano macho; plátano grande*
please	*por favor*
pleased to meet you	*mucho gusto; encantado/a*
plum	*ciruela*
pork chop	*chuleta de puerco; chuleta de cerdo; costillo de cerolo*

pork skins, fried	*chicharrones*
portion	*porción; ración*
potassium	*potasio*
potatoes	*papas; patatas*
pounds	*libras*
pregnancy	*embarazo*
pregnant	*embarazada*
prepared	*preparado/a*
pretzel	*prétzel*
problems	*problemas*
protein	*proteína*
pudding	*pudin*
pumpkin	*calabaza*
pumpkin seeds	*pepitas*

Q

quarter	*cuarto*
quarter past	*y cuarto*

R

raisins	*pasas; pasas de uva*
raw	*crudo/a*
relative	*familiar*
renal disease	*enfermedad renal; enfermedad de los riñones*
rice	*arroz*
rice, brown	*arroz integral; arroz moreno*
rice, white	*arroz blanco*
rice, wild	*arroz silvestre; arroz salvaje*
rice pudding	*arroz con leche*
rice water	*horchata; agua de horchata*
roasted	*asado/a*

S

salad	*ensalada*
salad dressing	*aderezo; aliño; condimento*
salt	*sal*
salt-free	*sin sal*
saltines	*galletas saladas*
sandwich	*sándwich; torta; bocadillo; emparedado*
saturated fat	*grasa saturada*
sausage	*salchicha; chorizo*
sautéed	*sofrito/a; salteado/a*
see you later	*hasta luego; hasta la vista*
see you soon	*hasta pronto*
see you tomorrow	*hasta mañana*
served	*servido/a*
serving	*ración; porción*
shellfish	*mariscos*
sherbet/sorbet	*sorbete; helado de nieve; helado de agua*
(I) should	*debo*
(you) should	*debiera*
skim	*descremado/a*
sliced	*rebanado/a; tajado/a*
slowly	*despacio*
small piece(s)	*trocito(s); pedacito(s)*
smoothie	*licuado*
snack	*merienda; bocadillo; entrecomidas*
sodium	*sodio*
soft drink	*refresco; gaseosa; soda*
soft drink, diet	*refresco dieta; gaseosa dieta; refresco lite; gaseosa lite*
so-so	*así, así; más o menos*
soul loss	*susto*
soup	*sopa*
spaghetti	*espaguetis; espaguettis*
Spanish	*español*
spices	*especias*
spinach	*espinacas; espinaca*
spread	*untado/a*
steak	*bistec; bife*
steamed	*cocido/a al vapor*
stewed	*guisado/a*
stir-fried	*sofrito/a*
strawberries	*fresas; frutillas*
strip(s)	*tira(s); rodaja(s)*
sugar	*azúcar*
sugar-free	*sin azúcar*
sweet(s)	*dulce(s)*
sweet potatoes	*batatas; camotes; boniatos*
syrup	*almíbar; sirope*

T

tablespoon	*cucharada*
(I) take	*tomo*
(to) take	*tomar*
(you) take	*toma*
tangerine	*mandarina*
tea	*té*
teaspoon	*cucharadita*

thank you	*gracias*
thirst	*sed*
(I'm) thirsty	*tengo sed*
(you're) thirsty	*tiene sed*
time	*tiempo*
to	*a*
toast	*pan tostado*
toast, wheat	*pan de trigo tostado*
toast, white	*pan blanco tostado*
toast, whole grain	*pan integral tostado*
tomato	*tomate; jitomate*
tomato juice	*jugo de tomate; jugo de jitomate*
tomato sauce	*salsa de tomate; salsa de jitomate*
tomorrow	*mañana*
too much	*demasiado/a; excesivo/a*
tortilla	*tortilla*
tortilla, corn	*tortilla de maíz*
tortilla, flour	*tortilla de harina*
tuna	*atún*
turkey	*pavo; guajolote*

U

unsaturated fat	*grasa no saturada; grasa insaturada*
usually	*usualmente*

V

vegetable juice	*jugo de verduras; jugo de vegetales*
vegetables	*verduras; vegetales*

very	*muy*
vitamin(s)	*vitamina(s)*

W

waffles	*wafles*
walnuts	*nueces de Castilla; nueces; nueces de nogal*
water	*agua*
watermelon	*sandía; patilla*
week	*semana*
(I) weigh	*peso*
(you) weigh	*pesa*
weight	*peso*
(not very) well	*(no muy) bien*
well-done	*bien hecho/a; bien cocido/a*
what	*qué*
What is your name?	*¿Cómo se llama usted? ¿Cuál es su nombre?*
when	*cuándo* (when asking a question); *cuando* (when making a statement)
where	*dónde* (when asking a question); *donde* (when making a statement)
whole grain	*integral*
whole wheat	*de trigo*
why?	*¿por qué?*
why not?	*¿por qué no?*
wine	*vino*
wine, red	*vino tinto; vino rojo*

wine, white	*vino blanco*
with	*con*
with less salt	*con menos sal*
without	*sin*

Y

yams	*batatas, camotes; boniatos*
years	*años*

yes	*sí*
yogurt	*yogur*
you	*usted*

Z

zucchini	*calabacita; calabacín; zapallito*